Great Sex after 40

Strategies for Lifelong Fulfillment

Marvel L. Williamson, Ph.D., R.N.

John Wiley & Sons, Inc.

New York • Chichester • Weinheim • Brisbane • Singapore • Toronto

To my husband, Paul,

who has never let me feel satisfied being less than I could be,

but who has always accepted me as I am

Published by John Wiley & Sons, Inc.
Published simultaneously in Canada

The information contained in this book is not intended to serve as a replacement for professional medical advice. Any use of the information in this book is at the reader's discretion. The author and the publisher specifically disclaim any and all liability arising directly or indirectly from the use or application of any information contained in this book. A health care professional should be consulted regarding your specific situation.

Library of Congress Cataloging-in-Publication Data

Williamson, Marvel L.
    Great sex after 40 : strategies for lifelong fulfillment
        p.   cm.
    Includes index.
    ISBN 0-471-35153-9 (pbk.)
    1. Sex instruction. 2. Middle aged persons—Sexual behavior. 3. Hygiene, Sexual. I. Title: Great sex after forty. II. Title.

HQ31.W754 2000
306.7'084'4—dc21   99-057415

Printed in the United States of America

10 9 8 7 6 5 4 3 2 1

CONTENTS

PREFACE

It all began in Mrs. Kavanaugh's fourth-grade class at Valley Falls (Kansas) Grade School. The boys had been sent out to recess while we girls sat in a darkened classroom and watched a film on menstruation. Afterward, the boys begged us to tell them about what they'd missed, but no one would—except me. Behind the countertop dividing the coat racks from the desks, I gathered a group of boys on the floor around me and launched into my first lecture on sex. It was an exhilarating experience. My audience transformed from a rowdy bunch of gigglers who at first couldn't believe what I was saying into my very own eager group of students full of questions. I was hooked. I never lost that wonderful feeling of fulfillment that comes from empowering others through the sharing of information. And I discovered that accurate sexual information was especially scarce.

Years later, the first graduate school course I took was on sexuality for health professionals. I was amazed at how much I learned from that simple course, which should have been included in my undergraduate nursing curriculum. Even today, new nurses and physicians continue to be undereducated about sexuality. My primary goal as a sexologist and as a professional Registered Nurse has been to fill this gap. I have taught thousands of nursing, medical, and other students of health care the basics of sexuality, how to assess patients for sexual problems, and techniques for treatment and referral. One of the problems preventing adequate sexual care is a lack of interdisciplinary communication and referral between the fields of sex therapy and clinical nursing or medicine. Another obstacle is the predominant attitude that as we age, sexual demise is normal.

Sexuality is an integral part of lifelong existence—the desire for sex doesn't stop when child-rearing days end. Human sexuality has no upper age limit. Unfortunately, many couples give up on sex when age-related physical changes and illnesses appear, either because they're too embarrassed to get help or because no one seems to have any solutions. The personal accounts in this book are composite summaries from my patients, where all identifying information has been changed to protect confidentiality. These stories represent the struggles of real people with sexual problems just like you may have experienced. The good news is that a couple can remain sexually active indefinitely if they work together to solve sexual challenges and have the right information on how to preserve sexual function.

My colleagues from health care, marital counseling, and sex therapy have asked that I write this book on how to adapt to sexual aging and illness. They are frustrated by the dearth of practical information, particularly for their clients/patients who misinterpret normal changes of sexual aging, as well as those who feel discouraged and uninformed about how to survive sexually through health crises.

My own clients/patients and lay audiences often tell me how hard it is to find accurate sexual information related to diseases and medical treatments. The stores are full of books on how to find love, how to improve a sexual or marital relationship, how to communicate better with a spouse, how to look sexier, and how to grow old "gracefully." But they can find nothing of substance on the unique problems of *sexual aging* and how age-related illnesses can affect sexual function.

Therefore, this book explains to anyone lucky enough to get older how to preserve and expand sexual capacity—no matter what. You see, this book was written for you.

ACKNOWLEDGMENTS

I thank God for giving me the perseverance to bring this book to completion, for opening doors so that the goal could become a reality, and for creating the people who invented computers and word processing.

I thank my husband, Paul S. Williamson, M.D., for the time and effort he spent critiquing every word of this book, for his professional expertise and advice, for his emotional and financial support throughout this project, and for being the most loving, sexiest life mate I could possibly want.

My colleagues, students, and clients/patients have always been valuable resources for material, questions, examples, and motivation. To anyone who has ever worked with me, sat under my tutelage, or benefited from my care, thank you.

Thanks, too, go to my sons, Marcus and Sean, for tolerating my grouchiness when the writing became tedious for me. I have also deeply appreciated my brothers, Don, Leland, and Paul Ansley, and their families for their support of my projects that have sometimes amused, embarrassed, or made them proud.

My literary agent, Sheree Bykofsky, is a champion representative who really knows her profession. Her advice on how to modify my scientific writing style into something more suitable for public consumption was right on target.

1

SEXUAL SURVIVAL
IN PERSPECTIVE

Once upon a time an average woman and an average man fell pas-
sionately in love with each other. They married and lived happily
ever after, enjoying an exciting and cozy sexual relationship 1.5
times a week until they died in each other's arms at the age of
ninety.

A fairy tale, you say? Absolutely not! If your fantasy is to stay
sexually active until old age with your personal Prince Charming
or Cinderella, then this book is your fairy godmother, ready to tell
you how you can make your dreams come true.

There is nothing better than traveling through time with someone you love, and having the joy of a thriving sexual relationship
with that person until the end of life itself. But perhaps you've
started noticing that sex requires more effort than it used to. It
could be that satisfying sex is no longer simply a matter of getting the kids out of your hair and putting on some romantic music.

Even if your relationship is based on good communication and
compromise, you will need new strategies to survive sexually as
you get older. This book will reveal how to add years to your
sexual journey together, in spite of health and aging problems
that appear more often. We have less energy as the years go by,

and our bodies become less dependable. Physical breakdowns cause problems that are bad enough, but the sexual implications compound our anxieties and self-doubts. Furthermore, our children and society as a whole stop expecting us to be sensual and sexual. It's tragic when a couple abandons sexual activity before they really want to because of sexual frustrations related to aging.

Here are some questions that may come up:

- Your husband survives his heart attack, but will your sex life survive?
- Coping with cancer is hard enough, but what can you do about the side effects of treatments that complicate sexual problems?
- What if your wife loses her sex drive after a hysterectomy?
- Why is it more difficult for men more than forty years old to get erections as often as they did when younger?
- What do you need to know about prostate pain during sex?
- When sexual intercourse begins to hurt, how can you avoid developing a sexual dysfunction or giving up on sex entirely?
- What if arthritis becomes so severe that intercourse become impossible?
- What if your diabetes is making penile erection more difficult to achieve?
- Can you have sex while wearing a colostomy bag?
- Should you continue taking your medicine for high blood pressure if it is interfering with your erectile ability?

This book will answer these questions and more. Many solutions may be as simple as experimenting to find new intercourse positions so that old "trick knee" doesn't swell and hurt the next day after having sex. Other sexual solutions will require more information, creativity, or even professional intervention. The answers are on the way!

THE MYTHS OF SEX AND AGING

"Sex is for the young." That message seems to blare incessantly from television, magazines, and other media. There's so much propaganda out there that it's almost impossible to hear from real people who are growing older and are still very much interested in sex. In this supposedly enlightened age of sexuality, why does the archaic view that sex is only for the young persist? When is someone too old for sex? The fact of the matter is, we're never "too old" for sex, because age does not determine sexual capacity. We may have to overcome many hang-ups, though.

One hang-up is the notion that physical beauty is perfect skin, toned bodies, and lustrous hair. There is a disturbing movement away from valuing the individual person as a whole being, toward prizing transitory external mirages. This shift not only sanctions the ridicule of sex for us older folks, but society also laughs at sex for the ugly, the fat, the bald, and the disabled. The lucky few who have the genes to look younger longer or the financial freedom to buy cosmetic surgery are admired for how well they retain their sexual aura. The praise focuses on their youthful appearance, ignoring the fact that sexuality is an inherent human quality and a right regardless of age.

Many among the "youth and beauty cult" (such as advertisers, producers, and even the average person who buys into the myth) truly believe that older people simply cannot be sexy and shouldn't even try to be. The younger generations berate us as "dirty old men" or "cradle robbers" or "lechers" or sad caricatures trying to hang on to our youth. Sometimes our children, the health care system, or nursing homes take away our sexual rights by forbidding conjugal visits, not allowing passes to go home, opening closed doors without knocking, and placing residents on sedatives who make sexual overtures. Many younger people who do not accept that sexuality is ageless have the misconception that sex is too strenuous for older persons.

When Geoffrey had his heart attack about twenty years ago, we were shocked by how difficult it was to get straightforward information about resuming sex. The doctors acted like we were too old to be interested in sex anyway. The nurses were so protective and cautious even about such simple tasks as getting up to the bathroom, that Geoff started feeling like he was too fragile for sex after all. I was mad and frustrated, and just knew if he was going to be strong enough for a cardiac rehab program, he must surely have strength for sex, too. Eventually we got the go-ahead, but not without some uncomfortable moments and not without facing the attitude that we were too old and fragile for sex.

THE FACTS OF SEX AND AGING

According to census figures, life expectancy is now seventy-five years, compared with forty-seven years at the turn of the twentieth century. There are currently eighty-five million people in the United States above the age of forty. From 1990 to 2050 the over-sixty-five age group is projected to increase by 117 percent, to sixty-nine million people. Proportionally, the fastest-growing segment of the population is the over-one-hundred age group. The time has come to pay attention to the sexual needs of older people.

Many studies confirm that most older people can be and still are sexually active. Even several decades ago, a 1972 Duke University study found that more than 75 percent of men seventy to seventy-nine years of age have intercourse at least once a month. They also found that 37 percent of the men between sixty-one and sixty-five in their study had intercourse at least weekly. Only 10 percent of men from sixty-six to seventy-one years of age have no interest in sex. A study by researcher Clyde Martin in 1977 reported that married men sixty to sixty-four years of age have intercourse an average of three times a month and that seventy-five-to-seventy-nine-year olds average at least once a month.

The Duke University study also discovered that 13 percent of women have *more* interest in sex after menopause. The sex research pioneers, Masters and Johnson, confirmed this finding, and also reported that the cause for lack of sexual interest in older women they treated was an unstimulating relationship. Older women often reveal that their biggest obstacle to regular intercourse was lack of a sexual partner, since usually the husband dies before the wife. As women age and their partners die, they turn to masturbation with greater frequency than when they were younger.

A fairly good study in 1994 by Robert Michael and associates (but unfortunately only polled people up to fifty-nine years of age—there's that age prejudice again) said that in the fifty to fifty-nine age group, 89 percent of men and 70 percent of women stated they were still sexually active, a logical reflection of partner availability for each gender. This again affirms that women lose sexual partners to death more often than men do. The fewer men available as women age is apparently the more limiting factor—not how old they are.

But there's a new type of sexual revolution that the revolution of the 1960s didn't touch. Older people are speaking out to say that even though our bodies are aging, we still want and need sex. We are asking how to maintain our sexual abilities even when our bodies give us new problems to overcome.

> *Janice and I always have had great sex. About two years ago, though, we "hit a wall" when we both turned forty. All of a sudden everything started falling apart. I had to get bifocals, her hair started turning gray really fast, I got a touch of arthritis in my right hand, and we both started noticing that we couldn't do as much on Saturdays as we used to without spending the next day recovering. I'd never had any impotence, but suddenly after one particularly exhausting weekend I totally let Janice down. She said it was no big deal, but I was embarrassed. What seemed weird to me was that I was definitely in the mood, but just couldn't get the little guy to cooperate.*

WHAT YOU NEED FOR SEXUAL SURVIVAL

Three essential elements enhance the likelihood that your sexual relationship will survive into old age:

1. **You must want to remain sexually active.** Reading this book is a good sign that you've already met this requirement. If you and your spouse have lost sexual desire for each other, though, you should investigate this problem with the help of a marriage counselor, preferably one certified by the American Association for Marriage and Family Therapy (AAMFT) or a sex therapist certified by the American Association of Sex Educators, Counselors, and Therapists (AASECT). Your health insurance might even cover the cost. This book may also help you understand why sexual interest is lagging.
2. **Develop a relationship characterized by commitment, ever-growing intimacy, and trust.** The next section more fully explains these predictors of sexual longevity, but if your relationship is severely deficient in these factors you might also benefit from professional counseling.
3. **You must understand what is happening to your aging (and often ailing) body and learn how to maximize and preserve your sexual potential.** Disclosure of this informa-

tion is the primary purpose of this book. Chapter 2 answers questions about sexual changes that are part of normal aging and what to do about them. Chapters 3, 4, and 5 address age-related sexual dysfunctions. Chapters 6 through 10 deal with specific illnesses, surgeries, drugs, and other therapies affecting sexuality.

Be willing to talk to your partner about your frustrations and needs, and listen openly to his or her needs as well. Give yourselves permission to try recommendations found in this book and to create some solutions of your own. Likewise, feel free to discard any suggestion that doesn't fit your unique situation.

How Commitment, Intimacy, and Trust Improve Chances of Surviving Sexually

Commitment

Commitment is an often preached but valuable concept. It simply means that you and your spouse have decided to stay together regardless of how you feel during the ups and downs of life. Why is commitment important to sexual survival? The rationale is simple but critically important:

1. Growing old brings about increasingly complex physical problems.
2. Coping with such problems requires a sexual partner who is not only willing to put up with some inconveniences but is also willing to communicate on an extremely intimate level to accommodate his or her partner's new sexual needs and limitations.
3. Such pressures on the sexual relationship require a deep love and desire to stay with the sexual partner regardless of personal inconvenience.

Not all marriages exemplify this relationship. Moreover, some couples have made this covenant to each other without the legal contract of marriage. Nevertheless, the most likely setting for long-term sexual success is within marriage. It is within the marital union that two people have promised to love each other, in sickness and in health, till death parts them.

This strong commitment presents the best opportunity for sexual solutions to work. It is within a good marriage that you're more likely to experience the joy that comes from physically loving another person and being loved back. Sexual activity between two people in love is an outward expression of a deeper psychological, spiritual connection. As someone who has invested considerable time into learning your spouse's needs, you're a long-term, understanding partner who is more likely to protect that investment and work harder when increased effort is required.

Problems inevitably appearing with aging are intensely personal in nature. Not only does knowledge of each other achieved from a long-term relationship make it easier to overcome problems, but also you must be willing to try because you promised to stay with and love each other through the difficulties. Waiting for someone to work through feelings and physical changes and finally coming to readiness for new options takes patience and requires a mature relationship. However, *good married sex—cozy, exciting, loving sex—is worth working and fighting for*. As Bernie Zilbergeld, a renowned expert on male sexuality, said, "Marriage offers the maximum opportunity for maximum gratification."

Another reason why a committed relationship affords the best opportunity for sexual success is the comfort factor. Cozy sex—that peaceful, warm joy during and after sex between two people in love and relaxed with each other—is often absent outside of marriage.

> *My best friend is my husband. When we decided twenty-eight years ago that we wanted to go together through that country called Time, our adventure began as a simple joy ride. Our friendship deepened as struggles and thrills led to greater intimacy in many aspects of our relationship. One of those has been sexuality. The feelings we have toward each other during sex are so deep that they're hard to describe. There is such security and love and excitement and relaxation all at once. We continually learn more about each other's sexual needs and desires. Every discovery, every experiment (even the ones that fail) is such fun! I can't imagine having sex with anyone else. I don't want to. I like married sex.*

A couple like this will be more willing to work to keep the joy of cozy sex when health problems or aging threaten to end it. They will grieve together when they cannot solve their sexual problems. They will become frustrated and angry when they cannot find answers to sexual questions.

Intimacy

"Being intimate" is a euphemism for having sex, but intimacy is much more than genital contact. It is knowing your spouse's private thoughts and secrets, and sharing his or her most personal feelings. It involves seeing each other as you really are, good and bad, in a variety of situations. Intimacy proceeds only as fast as the one of you who is more hesitant is willing to let it.

Because of the many complex layers that make up a person, intimacy comes slowly. We are all still discovering for ourselves hidden aspects of our own psyches, our physical makeup, our spiritual needs, and our intellectual potential. It is impossible to ever finish the quest for intimacy in ourselves or in another person. Couples can purposefully work toward greater intimacy and trust, though, by sharing their feelings, memories, fantasies, fears, and goals.

This relates to Masters and Johnson's finding mentioned earlier that the primary problem of older women in sex therapy is lack of a stimulating relationship. As long as a couple makes new discoveries about each other and creates new sexual experiences together, the relationship is more likely to be stimulating.

> *Kathy and I thought we had established a meaningful level of intimacy with each other because we were having sex—after all, how much more intimate can two people get?! We had jumped right into having sex after only a couple of dates. We certainly thought we were intimate, but discovered after several years of marriage with the help of a counselor that we had skipped several steps of sexual discovery and disclosure. We learned that having an orgasm together didn't mean we had a clue about what each other's sexual needs, preferences, or feelings were. We had never really discussed what we found pleasurable or disgusting. We were having sex with each other, but were doing it based on our sexual experiences with other people, or on what we each felt inside our own heads but never checked out with each other. We were having sex based on generalizations we had heard, not on a relationship with a particular unique person.*

Sexual intimacy is easier to accomplish on a physical than on a psychological level. While some couples who came to maturity during and after the "sexual revolution" of the '60s have little difficulty asking for what they want to get their sexual needs fulfilled, many find it hard to say the words aloud. It may take you years of giving your wife clues before you finally get the courage to tell her you want her to kiss your penis. You may fear hurting your husband's sexual ego so much that you don't admit you've been faking orgasms because his sexual techniques aren't correct for your needs.

Therefore, the type of intimacy that helps sexuality survive into old age comes not from one physical act or within a short period of time. It's a process of discovery and gradually increasing comfort leading to disclosure of secrets and new discoveries. It's hard to believe that a man and a woman could marry, have children, live together for three decades, and still lack intimacy. That's what happens, however, when a couple doesn't talk about their sexual needs even though they've made babies together.

You can achieve intimacy in two ways. First, delve more deeply into your spouse's inner thoughts and feelings. Ask questions. Discuss issues. Explore new topics. Second, broaden intimacy by expanding and widening the scope of experiences you've had together. Horizontal intimacy comes as you share more failures, crises, and joys.

Trust

For a couple to be successful at sexual aging, they must develop trust in each other. Trust is difficult, however, without years of experience during which each mate has seen the other honor the relationship over and over.

The ability to say to your wife, "Will you work with me to help me overcome the trouble I'm having getting an erection?" shows trust. The ability to admit to your husband that you're having pain during intercourse is another disclosure that requires trust. It's hard to share sexual secrets because they are both embarrassing and risky—embarrassing because they are so deeply personal, and risky because your partner could ridicule you or turn away instead of responding with love and concern.

You and your spouse can't trust each other on demand. You each must earn it. When one of you breaks trust, you must earn it all over again if the relationship is to thrive. Perhaps you're distrustful because your partner revealed embarrassing sexual secrets about you to your friends. Maybe broken trust in a prior relationship resulted in destruction of your marriage because one of you violated the commitment and reconciliation failed (if you tried reconciliation at all). Half of first marriages and even more second marriages in the United States do end in divorce, often because of lost trust.

If your first marriage ended in divorce, you can learn to overcome distrustful feelings with a new spouse. Because of prior marital experience, you may find it easier the second time to proceed faster through levels of intimacy. However, you may hide portions of your inner self out of fear, because you lost trust in your first marriage (and now you know from experience that it can happen again). If you're among the many who remarried after being widowed, you may feel guilty when you share confidential information with your new spouse that in the past only your first spouse knew. Or perhaps you feel guilty when engaging in sexual activities formerly reserved only for your first spouse. Open communication can eventually overcome such issues.

SEXUAL MILESTONES AND ROADBLOCKS ON THE HIGHWAY OF MARRIAGE

Most marriages pass through predictable sexual stages. We can predict sexual problems to a certain extent as well.

Stage 1: Newlyweds (and all couples first establishing sexual intimacy)

The first problem you may have had was turning off the message tapes running through your head telling you that sex was wrong—at least wrong before marriage. The transition from sexual abstinence to sexual freedom is an anxiety-filled step. Pressure to have intercourse on the wedding night in a state of fatigue and excitement can set the stage for problems, whether the couple is in their twenties *or sixties*. This is especially true for couples who have not taken progressive steps into sexual intimacy leading up to intercourse during the engagement period.

Another nearly universal complaint at this stage centers around how different men and women are in terms of how quickly or how slowly they become sexually aroused and how long each gender takes to reach orgasm.

> *Sex was terribly frustrating for us for a long time. I'd get turned on at the drop of a hat and hard before she had her bra off. Waiting for her to catch up enough to be ready for intercourse was agony. Sometimes it would take thirty to forty-five minutes of foreplay for her to be wet enough to get my penis in. I'd come within a minute or so, and then she'd be mad because she wasn't near orgasm.*

Men's sexual drive is much stronger as young adults than women's. Men understand their genitals better at a younger age and know how to come to orgasm faster than women do. Men are more likely to have masturbated, which is both a blessing and a curse, because they have learned how to orgasm easily but have also developed a pattern of rapid orgasm.

Women seem designed to respond to physical stimulation more slowly. Not only is the vagina not lubricated enough for intercourse by the time the penis is erect, but also a woman isn't likely to reach orgasm through intercourse alone. Just as the penis needs stimulation for orgasm, so, too, does the clitoris. Intercourse—that is, stimulation of the vagina—doesn't produce female orgasm, just as scrotal stimulation doesn't produce a male orgasm. Intercourse has sensual pleasures for a woman, but by itself it doesn't constitute a totally satisfying sexual experience. Clitoral stimulation to orgasm takes longer—sometimes thirty to sixty minutes longer—than penile stimulation to orgasm. As a woman ages, the length of foreplay may shorten some.

Another problem is a clash between how often each spouse wants sex. While the male libido is strong and peaks in early adulthood, the female sex drive tends to be more moderate and peaks in the third decade of life. A loving couple will find ways to accommodate each other's needs through creative sexual techniques when one is not in the mood for sex, or by negotiating the frequency of intercourse.

Stage 2: Pregnancy

During the first three months of pregnancy, the wife feels tired and nauseated. During the last three months she is large and uncomfortable. Throughout pregnancy, the husband is unsure about the safety of intercourse. After delivery, the woman is too sore and too tired for sex for a few weeks. The baby cries just when things start to get cozy. Dad becomes frustrated and horny. Mom's breasts leak milk when she is turned on. She feels fat and ugly. They are both tired from being up with the baby during the night. It's no wonder that sex gets shoved toward the bottom of the list of priorities. However, intimacy and trust can grow if they remain committed, communicate their needs, and work to meet those needs in new and old ways.

Stage 3: Child Rearing

The most common complaints of child-rearing couples are lack of privacy and interruptions. Life with children is hectic. Many parents feel chronically tired and overextended. The sexual relationship can easily suffer if not well tended to keep romance alive. Couples who marry for the second time and who already have children face an even greater challenge as they try to simultaneously build a new marital relationship. The child-rearing years are exhausting, often forcing the marriage to get nourishment only from tiny pieces of time here and there. A husband and a wife must remember that they are the core of the family. After the children move out, they don't want to find that they've become strangers to one another. Making sex a priority can help maintain that sense of "we're in this together" and that someday life will become sane again.

Stage 4: The Middle Years

In the middle age years (roughly forty to sixty-five), the children are finally more independent. However, aging begins to be a factor. The wife's sexual confidence and libido have been stronger for a while now, but the husband may appear bored or "played out." He falls asleep during foreplay. He wonders if his sexual attractiveness to other women is waning. Sex may have become boring and routine.

Perhaps your bad sexual habits persist because you've never become sexually intimate enough with each other to communicate about sex, or fear how your efforts will be perceived. Perhaps you use the same sexual techniques over and over, even though your spouse doesn't like them or finds them annoying, because he or she has never asked you to do anything different. Maybe your spouse doesn't know something different to suggest.

Physical problems start to appear. The man's prostate hurts a little during ejaculation now and then. You both run out of energy earlier in the day. Unexpected pain and creaks in the joints become puzzling concerns. Friends start having heart attacks and getting cancer. Menopause looms ahead and can strike a hard blow to a woman and her feminine sexual self-image, even though she knows it's coming and most women don't have severe symptoms.

> *My mother went through menopause when she was in her late forties, so I figured I didn't have anything to worry about yet. After all, I was very motivated to stay in shape and hang on to what I had. I faithfully used my skin treatments and night cream, stayed out of the sun, and was a serious believer in taking vitamins. I looked good and was very proud of it. When I was forty-three, though, I started having episodes of getting really warm and perspiring when everyone else around me felt fine. It didn't happen very often (about once a week), so I ignored it—that is, until two nights in a row I woke up drenched in perspiration. I told my best friend about it and she said it sounded like menopause. I refused to believe it, but thought I'd ask my doctor. She ran a hormone test and told me I was in early menopause. I was depressed for a good three months. Even though I knew everyone dies, nothing had ever happened personally to me before to make me think that I wasn't going to go on living forever.*

Stage 5: The Older Years

The biggest sexual problem at this time of life is slower sexual responsiveness: diminishing stamina, longer refractory periods, softer erections, vaginal dryness, and other physical problems that will be more fully described in chapter 2. These signs of sexual aging begin to appear in the middle years, but become serious deterrents to sexual enjoyment for most couples in their eighties and older. Other factors caused by serious health problems make sexual perseverance a challenge.

Psychological challenges caused by retirement or declining health can affect self-worth so dramatically that sexual confidence disappears. Eventually you may have to care for your sick or dying spouse, making the roles of caregiver and lover seem incompatible. You may find yourselves separated for prolonged periods by hospitalizations or will have to live apart if one of you enters a nursing home. Finally, widowhood or widowerhood is the ultimate adjustment. None of these events signals that your sexual road is at a dead end. There are alternative routes to sexual fulfillment.

THE REWARDS OF SEXUAL AGING

Now that we have roughly mapped the trip through the sexual life span, let's put the journey into perspective. Every stage of life has sexual challenges and adjustments. Every stage has sexual casualties, but more are likely to occur as the years pass. Some couples become discouraged, lose their sexual relationship, and give up physical contact with each other. For too many, marriage then evolves into a siblinglike living arrangement, with separate bedrooms.

Sexual aging does not have to be like that. There are solutions to sexual problems. There is hope as long as you're willing to learn and experiment and keep a sense of humor. Sometimes sex can be even better than before because the quality of the relationship is more mature.

It is natural and predictable for sexual feelings and activities to change over the years. Occasionally we have to trade certain forms of sexual intimacy for others. Sometimes we have to function alone sexually for a while, if not permanently.

There are so many reasons to be optimistic, though. For example, most women think older men are better at lovemaking. Older men feel more relaxed, tend to be more experienced, and have better sexual control over the timing of their orgasms than young men do. It's tragic when men misinterpret the natural slowing of sexual response that occurs with age as sexual dysfunction. It can, instead, be a wonderful bonus.

The older woman has sexual advantages, too, because she's more comfortable with her sexuality, usually has more insight into her sexual needs, and may be better able to express them to her husband. She may be more open to new sexual techniques and stimuli than she was when she was younger, revitalizing a boring sex life by exploring new levels of intimacy.

The couple who marries later in life or for the second time can often bypass differences in level of sexual desire. They find they're more closely matched in sex drive and speed of arousal than young people are. Couples who remain together throughout life also find that their sex drives become more compatible as they age.

In spite of physical declines, the *very positive* gains of aging, about which we hear too little, can enhance sexual satisfaction. Rewards emerge from ever-growing trust and intimacy in the marital relationship and strengthening of the psychological relationship resulting from long-term commitment to another human being. Orgasms feel just as good at an older age and are more precious. Other forms of intimate physical contact can become as pleasurable as an orgasm. The sensual relaxation of a leisurely massage not only makes aging muscles feel better and improves circulation, it also enhances the quality of sex. Rediscovering daytime sex can be exhilarating—a treat younger working couples rarely enjoy. Unhurried lovemaking without children in the house is another priceless luxury you can reclaim more often later in life.

> *At the age of fifty-two I am thrilled with my sex life! Young people are so smug because they think they have the corner on sex, but I've found that real sex doesn't start until you grow old with someone. I sure know my Ned is hotter than ever! We are so much more relaxed with each other than when we first married. Then later it seemed like the kids just sapped everything out of us. Plus, it took me a good twenty years to get over my sexual hang-ups. It took Ned about the same amount of time to get control of his orgasms. We are now finally discovering the fun of sex in the kitchen, sex on lunch break, sex in the yard after dark—we're just plain discovering real sex, not that desperate, embarrassed, rushed artificial stuff that twenty-year-olds think sex is!*

Finally, there is nothing better than still having that special person at your side who is the one you want to go through time with, knowing that person cares, understands, and will work hard with you to make sex better for as long as possible. These are comforting facts that make your "golden years" a reality, not a euphemism.

2

ADJUSTING TO NORMAL SEXUAL CHANGES

I'm often surprised when I look in the mirror and see a strange woman there who looks like my mother, but knowing it has to be me, of course. The constant rediscovery of what I look like as I grow older brings out the emotions of both happiness and anger. I feel pleased because maturity has many rewards. It's a relief to have the problems of youth behind me. For example, it's comforting to know I can relax from pressures to pursue a perfect body—I'm now contented to have a semifunctional body! I have a less hectic life, a simpler list of responsibilities, and the joys of adult children. I also feel angry, though, because aging is beyond my control. A corner of my mind believes I ought to be exempt from this insidious process and denies the reality in the mirror.

You probably have similar feelings. It's ironic that while our bodies age, our minds still see life through young eyes. It's difficult to believe we're like everyone else—that we aren't immune to aging. There are no exceptions, though. Aging overtakes every one of us who is fortunate enough to continue to survive. Ironically, aging brings on changes that would constitute some horrible disease if they occurred in a twenty-year-old but that we must learn to accept and graciously endure.

Everyone wants to hang on to the good things of youth, particularly sexual abilities. We find that sexuality actually becomes more valuable as time passes. It verifies our desirability to someone and boosts our egos. It even becomes more fun and fulfilling as we gradually release many of the inhibitions of our younger selves.

> *As the years roll by, I find myself becoming more conservative politically and socially. Oddly enough, though, my sexual self is freer than ever. I guess it's because my wife and I haven't yet discovered the outer limits of our sexual adventure together. Every so often we'll try something new, read a sex manual, see a spicier movie, or ask each other a question we've never before imagined. We engage in lovemaking techniques that as newlyweds we were too embarrassed to consider. Maybe we were ultraconservative to begin with, but I'm glad it's turned out this way. Sex just gets better and better!*

THEORIES OF AGING

Why do we grow older? What is the science behind sagging skin, graying hair, slower muscles, and the breakdown of our bodies? The answer remains one of the great mysteries of life. Several ideas are currently under investigation.

DNA Damage

One theory says that DNA, that chemical code that programs each of our cells, suffers damage over time when it divides to make new cells. Every time the cell divides again, that defect is passed to new cells. Over time more segments of DNA mutate and lose their original programming. The damage keeps accumulating in new cells until eventually the body begins to deteriorate.

Planned Obsolescence

Another theory proposes that DNA can create new cells only a limited number of times. After that limit, the body shrinks as fewer cells divide.

Free Radicals

As the body uses oxygen and nutrients, the by-products from the chemical reactions are not completely absorbed or modified. These by-products, called free radicals (atoms missing an electron), go around looking for electrons they're lacking. They can take electrons from anywhere—even DNA in living cells. Substances that lower free radicals are called antioxidants, because oxygen molecules make up most of the free radicals in circulation. It's too early to tell whether antioxidants can make a person live longer, though. In the meantime it's probably worthwhile to eat a diet high in antioxidants, such as vitamins C and E.

Metabolism

Some scientists speculate that metabolism is similar to the caramelization process during cooking. As metabolism, particularly in warm-blooded animals, converts oxygen and food into energy, waste products not passed from the body are deposited in our tissues. Like the ash left after a fire or the caramelized bits left in the skillet after meat finishes cooking, remaining waste products consist mostly of carbon. Carbon deposits cause less efficient tissue function over time.

Related to this theory is another that says if we decrease metabolism by eating less, we can prolong life. Mice whose food intake is cut severely do have longer life spans. A diet very low in calories, however, is almost impossible to tolerate. Not only is it difficult to get all nutrients needed from so little food, but people also feel as if they are in constant semistarvation.

Herein lies a paradox. While decreasing metabolism seems to lengthen life, maintaining an active lifestyle with moderate exercise helps slow aging, particularly in relation to flexibility and strength. However, exercise increases the body's metabolic rate and speeds aging.

Hormones

Some people think that since the pituitary gland makes less growth hormone as the years go by, the secret to slowing aging is by taking human growth hormone. Positive preliminary results include increase in muscle size, some fat loss, and improved skin integrity. However, the three injections necessary per week cost up to twenty thousand dollars per year. Once a person stops taking it, the good it produces disappears quickly, returning the body back to the same state of aging where it would have been without the hormone. DHEA (dehydroepiandrosterone) and melatonin are two other hormones that some people swear reduce the speed of aging. As with human growth hormone, scientific research is lacking, however. Most physicians warn about bad side effects.

What about sex hormones to prevent aging? Estrogen for women going through and past menopause does have some important benefits, mainly in protecting bone strength and preventing heart disease. Testosterone may benefit both men and women by improving sexual desire if levels are low, but it does nothing to slow the aging process.

The Bottom Line

Nothing but death prevents aging. The most we can do at present is to prevent disease through healthy lifestyles, closely monitoring our bodies, getting regular physical examinations, and staying "young at heart." Try instead to maximize sexual potential as you age, take each change in stride, and adapt so sexuality can continue. To know how to adapt, let's first review what happens to the body as it ages.

HOW THE BODY CHANGES WITH AGING

Tissues of the body deteriorate in two primary ways: shrinking (atrophy) and wearing out from years of use. For example, joints become stiffer and painful because the cartilage between bones shrinks and wears away with time. Eventually bone is rubbing against bone. Muscles also shrink, as much as 1 percent every year after thirty-five years of age, particularly in people who lead a sedentary lifestyle.

Bones

Bones lose calcium with age. This is especially a problem for women past menopause who don't take estrogen and don't get enough calcium and vitamin D. Men also lose calcium from their bones until when in old age they catch up to women, having the same severity of osteoporosis (the condition in which bones become more porous and brittle as calcium diminishes). Fractures are more likely, especially of the hips, wrists, and spine.

Arteries

Arteries become thicker and stiffer. Cholesterol buildup narrows inner passageways, and calcium deposits in the walls make them less flexible. The heart pumps harder to push blood through, resulting in high blood pressure. If an artery narrows too much, little or no blood can travel through it, causing the tissue it supplies to die. If this happens in the heart, we call it a heart attack. If it happens in the brain, it's a stroke.

The Senses

The eyes are especially susceptible to aging. The lens can become cloudy, a condition called cataracts. Focusing becomes more difficult as muscles that contract the lens weaken and the lens becomes stiffer. People who've had a lifetime of exposure to the sun without eye protection are subject to macular degeneration, blindness in patches on the retina.

The senses of smell and taste remain strong in some people but not in others. Genetics and damage over the years in people repeatedly exposed to loud noises can diminish hearing. The sensation of touch becomes more of a problem for diabetics because they can't always tell when something harmful is happening to their skin unless they see it happening with their eyes.

Skin and Hair

Sunlight is the worst culprit for skin, causing wrinkles, "age spots" or skin discolorations, and even cancer. Connective tissue supporting structures under the skin deteriorates, causing the skin to sag. Smokers wrinkle more because nicotine constricts blood vessels providing nourishment to the skin. Genes determine baldness in men, occurring in patches (male-pattern baldness). Both men and women experience generalized hair thinning.

Muscles

Muscles shrink because the number of muscle fibers decreases with age. Muscles tire more quickly and have a decreased work capacity. Breasts and buttocks sag. The bladder drops farther as muscles weaken and ligaments stretch, especially in women who have delivered many babies, causing difficulty controlling urine flow. Incontinence (involuntary leakage of urine) is an embarrassing problem for some women as early as their forties and worsens with time. Pelvic muscle exercises, medications, or surgery can relieve some incontinence.

Brain

The brain grows until about fifteen to twenty years of age, remaining the same size until about age fifty, when it gradually loses up to 25 percent of its weight. Fluid replaces brain tissue as it shrinks within the skull. The brain remains active but reflexes and memory slow, particularly recent memory. The best way to prevent loss of brain function is to use it for intellectual activities, puzzles, brain teasers, creating, writing, and problem-solving. Senility and Alzheimer's disease are not part of normal aging. Most older people remain functional mentally until just shortly before death.

Kidneys and Lungs

The lungs and kidneys are probably the most fragile of all body tissues. They are responsible for removal of the body's waste products, a process that eventually takes a toll. The lungs also lose their ability to expand fully. Oxygen exchange becomes less efficient. The kidneys become less effective at removing wastes and medicines from the bloodstream.

Testosterone

Testosterone levels in men should stay within the range of normal throughout life, but more of it can become bonded to proteins. The remaining amount of "free testosterone" decreases, particularly after age sixty. The result is as though testosterone levels have actually decreased, accounting for the slight shortening of the penis and the decrease in body and pubic hair. Morning erections occur less frequently, and the testes soften and shrink. They don't stop producing sperm, though. While the sperm count may drop some, fertility continues throughout life.

Prostate

The prostate gland, a walnut-sized organ that sits just under the bladder in men, also changes with age by enlarging (see also chapter 7). Since the urinary tube from the bladder to the penis passes through the prostate, this gland starts to put pressure on the urine passageway. As a result, many men have difficulty starting urination and find that it becomes increasingly uncomfortable.

During orgasm the enlarged prostate may hurt with the spasmodic contractions of ejaculation. This is especially a problem for men who have orgasms infrequently. Because of the pain, they may avoid sex, making the prostate become even more swollen and painful during ejaculation. The cessation of nocturnal emissions as men age also contributes to prostate pain. In younger men, wet dreams act as a spontaneous release valve, so to speak, relieving pressure in the prostate when orgasms occur less often than needed as fluid accumulates.

Menopause and Beyond

Menopause is the permanent cessation of ovulation and menstruation caused by declining ovary function. It is completed when the last menstrual period occurred at least one year previously. Eggs diminish in number, and estrogen and progesterone dwindle. The average woman completes menopause at fifty to fifty-one years of age. Almost all have their last menstrual period by age fifty-five.

Menopause may cause hot flashes, unpredictable episodes of generalized warmth often starting in the face, neck, or scalp and spreading throughout the body. Hot flashes don't happen to every woman and are not dangerous, but can be embarrassing because they start without warning and cause such copious sweating. A woman suffers from such an intense feeling of heat that she can soak her clothes or bedsheets with perspiration. If hot flashes occur often during sleep, her mood will change and she will have less stamina because of severe sleep disturbances. Irritability or depression accompanying menopause can actually be due to a woman not getting enough sustained sleep every night.

> When I was only forty-one years old I began having hot flashes. At first I thought I was just "warm-blooded" because it seemed as if I was always hot when everyone else was cold. But then I started waking up at night, just radiating heat. Before I allowed myself to consider that it might be menopause, I spent a lot of time telling myself I was too young for "the change." By the time I decided to get help from my doctor, hot flashes were getting me up two or three times a night. Every time I had to change my nightgown and underwear, wash my face, air the bed, and cool off for a few minutes. During the days, I was a real witch. I thought it was because I was mad about getting older, but once I started on estrogen, the hot flashes virtually disappeared, I slept better, and my mood improved tremendously!

Decreasing estrogen causes several other changes throughout the body, too, because it's the primary hormone responsible for female physical characteristics. Estrogen turns a girl into a woman at puberty. Its disappearance at menopause reverses some of those changes. For example, breasts shrink some and the uterus loses about half its weight.

The lack of estrogen also has a profound effect on the vagina. The acidity of the vagina changes, making it more alkaline. The acidity keeps the microbes that normally live in the vagina under control, but after menopause they can start to grow too rapidly. Vaginal infections (vaginitis) can start more easily.

The vagina also loses some elasticity. Fat deposits around the vagina diminish, reducing some of its supple cushioning. The vagina becomes drier, especially five years following the last menstrual period. Dryness is a problem during sexual inter-course, but can also cause irritation and itchiness unrelated to infection. Some women mistakenly believe they have vaginitis, when their vaginas are merely dry and would benefit from artificial lubricants or estrogen cream.

> *I had had vaginitis only twice in my life, but when I hit forty-three it seemed as if I was getting an infection every two or three months! There wasn't really any cheesy discharge or odor, but my genitals burned and itched horribly. I faithfully used the yeast creams from the drugstore. I even started eating yogurt, a home remedy my best friend swore by for preventing infections. Nothing helped, though. Intercourse left me in agony. I was embarrassed and frustrated and finally saw my family doctor about it. She found no infection and said I was probably in early menopause. She prescribed estrogen cream to smear on my labia and to put into my vagina. In a couple of weeks, the soreness disappeared.*

Another effect of decreased estrogen is smoothing of the vaginal lining and decreased blood flow around it, particularly during sexual arousal. In younger women the vaginal lining has a corru-gated look. The ribbed appearance of the tissue (called rugae) be-comes flatter with age, possibly reducing friction on the penis during intercourse.

Menopause also causes vaginal atrophy (shrinkage). The lining of the vagina becomes thinner and less resilient, contributing even more to itching and irritation. Vaginal atrophy and dryness are less problematic in women who stay sexually active. Even masturbation of the clitoris can help preserve the vagina some because sexual arousal increases circulation to the tissues and helps keep them lubricated. Better than external masturbation is intercourse once or twice a week (or use of a dildo, an artificial penis or similarly shaped object inserted into the vagina), which helps slow vaginal atrophy more than anything else. The massaging effect on the tissues promotes circulation and improves tone. The penis keeps the vagina stretched, open, and resilient.

Aging also affects the length of the vagina. In the unstimulated state, the vagina of the young woman is about three inches long. A sexually inactive woman over sixty, however, has a vaginal length of about two inches. How much shorter the vagina gets with age is partly dependent on whether the woman is continuing to have intercourse regularly.

A woman past menopause who hasn't had intercourse for a long time must take special precautions if she plans to become sexually active again, typically a widowed woman who later remarries. Plunging right into intercourse could injure the thinner, atrophied vagina. She needs to start inserting estrogen cream into her vagina for at least two weeks before she resumes intercourse. If she begins estrogen pills or skin patches, she should wait at least four weeks before resuming intercourse.

It is also very important that a woman renewing sexual activity have a thorough vaginal examination to ascertain whether there are adhesions within the vagina. Adhesions (small connective bands of tissue) may have formed during sexual inactivity. A physician can release the adhesions without hospitalization. The woman should expect some slight vaginal bleeding after the procedure, but usually experiences little pain because the adhesions have no nerve supply. Another suggestion is to use a dildo during masturbation at least once before resuming intercourse, to stretch the vagina and become accustomed to the sensation of having something in it again. This will help alleviate fear of pain during intercourse.

> When Harry and I met, I had been widowed for eleven years and his Eleanor had been gone for four years. We were both awkward about "dating." Once we started, though, it was only a few weeks until we were so happily in love and grateful for each other's companionship that we got married. I had worried about having sex, but thought that love would conquer all. After all, my first husband and I had never had any problems. On our wedding night, Harry was very tender and careful. Eventually I started to feel my-

self respond. We tried to have intercourse for nearly an hour until I became so embarrassed that I locked myself in the bathroom in tears. Every time he had tried to enter me, it felt like something was blocking his way. After a while it started to hurt and I tensed up even more. We used Vaseline and even tried a couple of different positions, but nothing worked. A week later I finally gave in and let him take me to see a gynecologist. Snip, snip! was all it took! Looking back, I realize how foolish I was to try to have sex without a pelvic exam first.

All the conditions related to menopause can diminish greatly by taking estrogen pills, wearing a patch, and/or applying cream to the vagina and labia on a regular, ongoing basis. Estrogen replacement therapy should continue for the rest of your life. A woman several years past menopause who hasn't taken estrogen can begin even then and receive benefits.

Many years ago women feared that estrogen contributed to development of certain cancers, especially of the uterus lining (endometrial cancer) or breast cancer. Physicians now prescribe estrogen in lower doses and in combination with progesterone, another female hormone, to greatly decrease cancer risk. The benefits of estrogen for slowing heart disease and preventing osteoporosis greatly outweigh the much less common occurrence of cancer. Estrogen combined with continued sexual activity also provide the best antidotes to female aging, particularly aging of the genital and reproductive organs.

Don't Stop Reading Here!

The changes that come with aging could be discouraging, if that were the end of the story. They are manageable, though. Remember, good sex is worth the effort. Your body needs it, your mind needs it, and your spouse will treasure you for it. There is more than hope, there are solutions!

HOW SEXUAL RESPONSE CHANGES WITH AGING

Human sexual response involves the physical events during sexual arousal, orgasm, and recovery. William Masters and Virginia Johnson defined four stages of sexual response based on their pioneering research: excitement, plateau, orgasm, and resolution.

As sex therapists applied Masters and Johnson's research, it became apparent that not all sexual problems fell into those four phases, so the desire phase was added.

Desire Phase

Overview.   For sex to take place there must be willingness, interest, and attraction to someone. A healthy sex drive (libido) is an important factor in the desire phase. A lack of desire for sex may have nothing to do with libido, though. Perhaps you have a functioning sex drive but are simply too tired for sex sometimes. Circumstances have to be right. Stress, the wrong partner, the wrong timing, and other factors also can inhibit the ability to become sexually aroused. Sexual frustrations due to poor communication may kill the mood, sometimes making couples decide that the effort isn't worth the little pleasure it gives.

> *Janice never had been crazy about sex for some reason. She tried to please me, but it was obvious she wasn't getting much out of it. As we got older, she began to resist sex. She acted irritated whenever I showed any interest. When she did give in, she just lay there. I can't remember the last time she had an orgasm. After a while it took its toll on me. After all, what kind of guy would want to force himself on a woman who obviously wasn't interested? The less we had sex, the more I got used to having it less. After a few months, we stopped having sex altogether. The crazy thing is, we never even talked about it.*

Better communication by women could solve many of their frustrations, such as insufficiently long foreplay and improper stimulation of the clitoris.

Guilt feelings from almost anywhere can also kill sexual desire: extramarital affairs, engaging in masturbation, "wild" fantasies, family problems, or just bad feelings about enjoying sex. Fear of sex destroys desire, too. Fear can develop from being sexually assaulted, believing myths about sex, having surgery or a heart attack, feeling anxiety about getting AIDS, having sexual "hang-ups," or a multitude of other possibilities.

These emotions and others create a physiological conflict. The "fight or flight" response controlled by one part of the nervous system (the "sympathetic system") prevents sexual arousal, which is under the control of the parasympathetic nervous system. Fear and arousal usually cannot occur simultaneously.

Given the right circumstances, though, sexual desire in a healthy adult works properly if the opportunity for sex exists. A normal sex drive in both men and women depends in part on the influence of testosterone. The testes make testosterone in men, and the ovaries and adrenal glands make lesser amounts of it in women.

Age-related changes in women.   Women who lose their desire for sex as they age usually do so as a result of circumstances or psychological factors, not physical. For example, some women believe menopause means the end of sexual activity because reproduction ceases. In their minds, sex and reproduction are one and the same. If they assume sex no longer has a purpose, they lose their desire for it—especially if they never received much pleasure from it anyway. For others, menstrual irregularities during menopause alter sexual patterns and hinder spontaneity.

> *I don't think men have a clue about what women go through during menopause! They know about hot flashes and mood swings, but understanding what it's like to never know when a period is going to start has to come from experience. Forget the calendar! Forget that you just had a period last week! You never know when one is going to hit or how long it'll last. And sometimes it's a real "gusher." I always wear a pad whether I'm on a period or not, having learned the hard way. And then my husband wonders why I'm not as spontaneous sexually as I used to be! I never was one for liking sex during my period anyway, and now I never know when the next one is coming. I finally decided to pull out an old diaphragm I had kept. Whenever it looks like he's interested in having intercourse, I put the diaphragm in to stop the blood flow and wash off real well. If I read him wrong, I just take it out later and clean up the mess. It's a hassle, but it's okay temporarily.*

Some women use menopause as an excuse to have sex less frequently, particularly if it wasn't satisfying before menopause. *The best way to predict how much people will enjoy sex later in life is to look at how much they enjoyed sex when younger.* Husbands whose wives claim that they've lost their interest in sex because of menopause should gently discuss their sexual relationship frankly. Professional counseling helps, too.

Sometimes loss of sexual desire after menopause is due to

pain during intercourse, which is very treatable, but aging itself shouldn't diminish sexual desire. In fact, *sexual desire may increase after menopause* because as estrogen decreases, the effect of testosterone may strengthen. The ovaries don't stop producing testosterone. When younger, estrogen overwhelmed the small amount of testosterone, but after menopause that effect switches. Many women also have stronger sex drives after menopause because they feel freedom from getting pregnant and having to use birth control.

Another factor can be because our society puts such high value on physical beauty and youth. It's difficult for women to retain their self-esteem when their skin sags, they gain weight, buttocks dimple and drop, and other changes become apparent. Men have such feelings much less often and may be unaware how significant these changes are to women. A wife is very vulnerable to her husband's comments about how she looks. She may start to avoid being nude around him and hide under the covers or in the dark during sex.

Marilyn had always been my little nymphet. She loved to do a slow striptease for me. Our sex life was great—until a few weeks ago, that is. I didn't notice for quite a while that she'd become more modest, but one morning she really blew up at me when I walked in on her while she was still bathing. It took several days of this before I realized I hadn't seen her naked in a long time. The next time we made love I tried to be subtle about it and kept the lights on low to see what would happen. She turned them off. I began to tease her about what she was hiding, and before I knew it she was sobbing about how ashamed she was. Apparently a few weeks earlier she'd had occasion for the first time in a long time to look at her naked backside and was horrified to see how dimpled and saggy it had become. I couldn't bear to tell her I'd noticed that starting to happen ten years ago, but did have the brains to convince her that what was sexy about her was the feminine shape of her body—not her muscle or skin tone. We finally were able to laugh about it, as I pointed out my own paunch and sagging buns, which she admitted didn't bother her diddly. She's been my little nymphet again ever since.

Obviously there are many reasons why a woman may lose desire for sex as she ages. *The number one factor has to do with her* lack of a sexual partner, though, not loss of physical ability or poor self-image. If sex is not available to her, she may eventually lose interest in it. Even if her husband is still around, *he* may have lost interest in sex or failed to adjust sexually when a serious illness hit.

If a couple stops having sex, it's usually because of erectile failure or illness of the husband. This reflects the fact that in most relationships men initiate sexual activity more often than women. Perhaps related to this, women masturbate more frequently after menopause than before, an alternative every woman should feel free to explore because of its important physical benefits (e.g., improving circulation to the pelvic organs, lubricating dry vaginal tissues to prevent vaginitis, and preserving the openness of the vaginal passage).

Age-related changes in men. The sexual drive peak drifts further into the past, but the *quality* of sexual experiences usually improves for men. As the male ego becomes linked less to sexual prowess, it identifies more with career and other successes. The quality of sex also improves because male and female sexual response rates become more compatible.

On the other hand, diminished sexual desire correlates with occasional episodes of sadness when events related to career or other factors cause a man to confront his shrinking future, dissatisfaction over lack of accomplishments, and diminishment of self-esteem if he believes his usefulness is declining.

> Jerry was forced into early retirement last year. He was bravely cheerful about it to everyone else, but at home alone with me he was depressed. He talked about being just an old shoe that had gotten thrown away when it wore out. He didn't want to do anything, especially have sex. He began to scare me with his talk about having no future. With the help of one of his best friends, I got him to see a doctor, who gave him an antidepressant and referred him to a cognitive therapist. It has really made a huge difference in his outlook, and now sex is back on track.

As long as a man remains healthy, there should be no physical reason for him to lose his sex drive. This is true even though men normally produce slightly less amounts of testosterone over the years until about age sixty, when it stabilizes. If sex drive loss is severe, it is worthwhile to see a physician and request testosterone-level tests, particularly to distinguish between the amount of (usable) "free" versus "bound" testosterone in circulation.

A physician may not recommend testosterone replacement therapy, though, because it promotes atherosclerosis (hardening of the arteries) and prostate tumors. However, the cause of low testosterone may itself be reversible, bringing about renewed sexual desire. Causes of dropping testosterone levels are pituitary or hypothalamic tumors or diseases (particularly prolactin hormone-secreting tumors), thyroid deficiency, liver disease, and estrogen-secreting tumors.

Men are much more likely to lose sexual desire from excessive alcohol and food than from low testosterone. Both substances numb the senses and slow the body. Alcohol also causes erectile dysfunction. In fact, alcohol abuse causes more erectile failure between forty-five and fifty-five years of age than any other factor. If alcohol abuse continues, liver damage results, which in turn can cause testicular shrinkage and male breast enlargement.

Age-related changes in both men and women. Another cause of lost sexual desire is high-level tension and chronic stress that may accumulate with age, temporarily lowering testosterone in both genders by the effect of stress on the adrenal glands, which in turn affects the hormonal balance of the endocrine system. Most illegal drugs and some medications also knock out sexual desire or function, such as blood pressure medicines, some psychiatric drugs, and sedatives (tranquilizers).

Interest in sex does not normally go away with simple aging, however. Sexual interest decreases far more slowly than sexual activity. If there are no apparent physical, psychological, or relationship problems, your loss of sexual desire may be due to something as straightforward as a dull, boring, and routine sex life that uses the same lovemaking techniques over and over. Perhaps desire is waning because your relationship with your spouse hasn't deepened in spite of the years together. You are no closer to sexual intimacy and know little about each other's sexual needs.

We're pretty typical. At least that's what I pick up from our friends and TV. Everyone always hears the jokes about how monotony and monogamy are the same thing—right? Well, that sure fits us. Sex was great for the first three years or so, but twenty years later it's only one step better than a chore. Every time it's the same thing: Saturday night after the late news, same format, same position, same little squeeze afterward, and a quick "Love you, too" before the snoring starts.

Fortunately, the ability to renew sexual interest and revitalize lovemaking is absolutely possible. Even widows and widowers more than eighty years of age have a dramatic rise in sexual interest when they fall in love with someone new. Read a book together, such as one from Alex Comfort's *Joy of Sex* series, to get ideas about ways to put the spice back into a bland, boring sex life. Refocus sexual pleasuring away from orgasm and intercourse and toward sensual stimulation. Rebuilding the marriage (especially after the last child leaves home) improves sex. Pursuing recreational activities together, rediscovering companionship, and sharing humor renew sexual feelings, too.

Techniques used by counselors and leaders of marriage encounter weekends can also reestablish communication and promote intimacy. While it's not the purpose of this book to get into marriage therapy, simple exercises can add a new spark of sexual desire by improving your communication. For example, you can each separately write a list of your apprehensions and hopes related to your sexual relationship. Share your lists and discuss them seriously. Another activity is to complete the exercise in chapter 4 to broaden sexual techniques. Periodically add new topics to your discussions to aid the discovery and sexual renewal process, such as how to communicate to your spouse you're interested in having sex. Another discussion could deal with what to do when one of you wants sex but the other doesn't. Is masturbation acceptable, or are you willing to help each other have an orgasm through manual or oral stimulation? Such discussions not only heighten sexual desire and interest in intimacy, they also improve marital communication by eliminating guesswork.

Excitement and Plateau Phases (Arousal)

Overview. The second phase of human sexual response is excitement, during which changes begin to occur from physical or psychological sexual stimulation. The third stage, "plateau," is an advanced stage of excitement when physical tension continues to grow and persist for a while prior to orgasm. These stages together make up sexual arousal.

Sexual arousal results from two primary phenomena. The first, *vasocongestion* (swelling of vessels and tissues with blood), explains genital enlargement. As blood flow increases and becomes trapped in the special spongy cavities designed to fill during sexual activity, the penis and the clitoris become larger, longer, firmer, and stand away from the body in erection. The vagina expands and lengthens as well. The genitals become warmer and redder. Vasocongestion also expands the skin folds (labia) on either side of the clitoris and vaginal opening, causing them to flare open, making the vaginal entrance more visible.

Vasocongestion affects internal organs, too. The size of the testes increases and the uterus swells slightly and tilts higher into the abdomen. The nipples become erect. Women's breasts also swell. Many people acquire a "sex flush," a splotchy redness over the skin that usually starts on the chest and spreads to the neck.

Vaginal lubrication results from moisture seeping through the vaginal wall as blood flow increases. Lubrication is important, not only because it signals that a woman is becoming sexually aroused, but also because intercourse hurts her if the vagina isn't slippery enough. Blood flow around the vagina also enlarges the "orgasmic platform," the outer third of the vagina, creating a tighter grip on the penis. The prostate gland also swells. While the prostate makes most of the ejaculate fluid, the Cowper's gland secretes a preorgasmic fluid that oozes from the tip of the penis and may contain sperm, too.

The second phenomenon during sexual arousal is *myotonia*, an increase in muscle tension. Myotonia appears in the genitals as a tightening of the male scrotum, pulling the testes closer toward the base of the penis. Muscle tension also occurs in the arms, legs, hands, feet, and facial muscles, shown by how much tighter and rigid they become. Other changes during arousal include elevations in blood pressure, heart rate, and breathing rate.

Many women describe a sensation during arousal called a "vaginal ache," essentially a physiologically based desire for intercourse, due to the spreading open of the uppermost portion of the vagina near the cervix (the opening of the uterus). This "tenting effect" is described by some women as an empty feeling deep inside the vagina, others as an intense need for penile pressure.

The length of the excitement and plateau stages differs for each gender. If a man begins stimulating his penis and a woman her clitoris at the exact same time and try to achieve orgasm simultaneously (not a valuable goal, by the way), the man's excitement phase is shorter. His plateau phase would then have to be longer as he waits for the woman to catch up. In other words, arousal occurs more rapidly for men than for women.

> *Lana and I used to believe that successful sex meant we would have our orgasms at the same time. Maybe that sounds a little crazy, but we got that idea from the movies. We saw the same thing over and over—the couple on the screen was obviously having their orgasms simultaneously in a grand climax of passion. We valiantly tried to do the same for years and finally gave up in frustration. It was the smartest thing we ever did. Now we can concentrate on each other's orgasm. I can make sure her clitoris gets the attention it needs (something I always had trouble doing while trying to come myself). Plus, Lana is always much more lubricated after her orgasm, which makes intercourse more comfortable for her when I'm ready to focus on it being my turn.*

It's difficult to overemphasize the importance of clitoral stimulation. Without it both partners can become frustrated over how long it takes the vagina to become adequately lubricated and how long it takes a woman to achieve orgasm. In fact, she usually cannot reach orgasm at all solely through intercourse.

Age-related changes in women. The number one problem as women age having to do with sexual arousal is inadequate vaginal lubrication following menopause. This is a direct result of decreased estrogen, but can be prevented or reversed by estrogen replacement therapy.

Decreased engorgement affects both genders. As the years pass, artery walls become harder and expand less efficiently. Buildup of cholesterol plaque inside the arteries narrows them, reducing blood flow to genital and pelvic tissues. Although the clitoris, labia, and orgasmic platform engorge less, most women say their vaginas continue to provide adequate pressure on the penis during intercourse. Breasts do not swell as much. The uterus does not enlarge and, as time goes by, elevates less into the abdomen during arousal. The tenting effect may not appear until late in the plateau phase and then to a lesser extent. Vasocongestion as manifested by the sex flush becomes less prominent in both men and women with age.

Age-related changes in men.   Atherosclerosis of deep arteries can cause decreased penile vasocongestion. Erections are softer. The penis "stands up" less, also because ligaments that suspend the penis lose their elasticity. Furthermore, shrinkage of muscles on the floor of the pelvis contributes to less rigidity of the penis.

> *I honestly thought I was becoming impotent. When I was seventeen I remember having real hard-ons in a flash from just seeing a sexy girl on the street. When I was in my late twenties, I began noticing that even though I was still willing and ready, my little soldier didn't stand at attention as much as it used to. My wife didn't seem to notice, and I tried not to think about it. In my thirties, my erections were just a little softer, but still I figured it was no big deal. In my forties, I really started getting worried. Not only was I even a little softer, I got hard less often when seeing a sexy woman. I didn't get fully erect until during sex, when my wife started foreplay with me. Sex still felt great, but I was worried. At my physical checkup I asked my doctor about it, and he said I was perfectly normal—all guys go through this. That really blew my mind, but it's great to know there's nothing wrong.*

With age, erections gradually take longer to achieve. Men require more direct stimulation of the penis, and are unable to acquire the full and automatic erections that young men have just by thinking about sex. The need for physical stimulation for erections may begin as young as forty years of age, but is characteristic of most men by age fifty. Full erection does not become complete until just prior to orgasm. The testes also change. Due to diminished vasocongestion, decreased muscle tone, and thinning of the scrotal skin, they elevate and enlarge less.

It's easy to misinterpret these changes. Many of us mistakenly believe we are losing our sexual abilities. It's not surprising that a man who has always had little difficulty obtaining fast, hard erections by just thinking about sex would worry when he gradually loses this ability. Such anxiety can cause erectile dysfunction, though, contributing to depression and loss of interest in sex.

Some men concerned about losing their potency protect themselves by avoiding all sexual contact. They stop showing affection, dreading that their wives will misinterpret it as a desire for sex. Their wives don't understand what has happened and may believe their husbands no longer love them, no longer find them sexually desirable, or are having an extramarital affair. Sometimes men withdraw from sexual contact, fearing they may discover further loss of function, or feeling embarrassed about their softer erections. Their wives may even have commented unkindly and mistakenly about "impotence," also unaware that the changes observed are normal and that orgasms are still possible.

Women are vulnerable to self-doubts, too, as they notice changes in their own bodies. All people who feel embarrassed about their aging bodies and abilities risk loneliness and bitterness if they withdraw from sexual contact, though, and their spouses will feel rejected. If a couple cannot talk to each other to talk about these challenges, they need marital counseling to salvage their sexual relationship.

Orgasm Phase

Overview.   As the peak of sexual fulfillment both physically and emotionally, orgasm is a very pleasurable experience involving release of muscular tension as nerve impulses fire, causing a shuddering (almost seizurelike) response. The sensation is similar for both sexes. The main difference is the ejaculatory experience for men, and the possibility of prolonged or multiple orgasms for women.

For orgasm, stimulation of the penis or clitoris is essential. (In certain circumstances people can learn to orgasm through stimulation of other body parts, but usually only after learning how to reach orgasm through penis or clitoris massage first.) Discovering how to orgasm is harder for women than for men. Self-education through masturbation helps immeasurably. Shere Hite's extensive research found that the number of women who have never experienced orgasm is five times higher among those who have never masturbated.

About half of all women occasionally pretend to have orgasms. While it's difficult for men to fake erections, men, too, can fake orgasms—especially during intercourse. Habitual faking signals a need to communicate regarding the type of sexual stimulation needed, or may signal that the couple needs therapy for sexual dysfunction.

Not all women are capable of multiple orgasms, and those who are not shouldn't feel cheated. A single orgasm is just as pleasing. A multiple orgasm is two or more orgasms in rapid succession, or one prolonged orgasm lasting for more than 20 seconds. Multiple orgasms occur only in women because female sexuality doesn't include a refractory period (see "Resolution Phase" later in this chapter).

During orgasm both genders experience contractions in their genital areas and rectal sphincters (the tight band of muscles around the anal opening). Contractions occur at 0.8-second intervals, lasting 3 to 10 seconds for men and 3 to 20 seconds for women. Women feel the spasmodic contractions throughout their orgasmic platform (the outer third of the vagina), the urinary tube, and the uterus—particularly if they are pregnant.

Men orgasm in two stages. The first is "ejaculatory inevitability." For 2 to 4 seconds just prior to semen release, men feel that ejaculation is about to happen and that they cannot stop it. This sensation results from contractions along the organs of their internal semen pathway, putting the ejaculate fluid under pressure inside the urinary tube just below the bladder within the prostate. The semen doesn't enter the bladder because the internal sphincter (muscle that stops urine flow out of the bladder) closes during erection.

The second stage of male orgasm is ejaculation. The prostate, urinary tube, and rectal sphincter contract. The ejaculation of semen in spurts from the tip of the penis corresponds to the 0.8-second-interval contractions. Men can feel the ejaculate fluid passing through the urinary tube with so much pressure that in young men it spurts out 1 to 2 feet from the penis.

Both genders experience mild loss of control as leg muscles and other body parts spasm involuntarily during orgasm. The heart rate continues to accelerate to as high as 160 to 180 beats per minute. Breathing increases to 40 breaths per minute.

Age-related changes in women.   As people age, the quality of orgasms doesn't diminish. However, some changes can be worrisome. For example, postmenopausal uterine contractions during orgasm and for up to a minute after can hurt, as if the uterus were irritated. Estrogen replacement therapy helps prevent uterine pain during orgasm.

Women capable of multiple orgasms retain that ability throughout life. They may find that orgasm during every sexual encounter is less important as time passes. Intercourse takes on more purpose than simply achieving an orgasm—such as fun and fulfillment, affection, companionship, attention, and sharing intimacy.

Intercourse also feels good with or without orgasm for women who have learned how to use the PC (pubococcygeus) muscles. These muscles, at the outer third of the vagina, can be identified by noticing which muscles start and stop urine flow. By tightening them during intercourse, a woman can grip the penis more tightly and enjoy heightened erotic sensations in the vagina.

> *When I learned how to tighten my PC muscles during sex, I discovered a whole new level of sexual ecstasy. I don't know why, but if I'm not feeling particularly aroused, just by squeezing down on my husband's penis with my PCs boosts my arousal tremendously. It's opened a new dimension of pleasure.*

Age-related changes in men. One benefit of aging is that any tendency toward premature ejaculation fades. As men age they gain better control over their orgasms, making them better lovers.

The two-stage process of male orgasm melds into a single ejaculatory process over the years. The sensation of impending orgasm may decrease in duration to just a second or so (although some men describe a prolonged ejaculatory inevitability phase). Contractions of the prostate during ejaculation may diminish. If the prostate is enlarged, there can be pain during orgasm. Ejaculation is less forceful, characterized by one or two gentle waves. Since there is less internal pressure, seminal fluid may seep out or spurt a shorter distance than when younger.

Because of muscle shrinkage in the pelvis and rectal sphincter, and possibly less free circulating testosterone, muscle contraction strength during orgasm diminishes a little. This partially accounts for the decrease in ejaculation force and potential disappearance of rectal sphincter contractions in men over fifty. Ejaculate fluid volume decreases slightly. Sperm production continues, although the sperm count may be somewhat lower.

Having an ejaculation or expelling semen is not necessary to male orgasm. In fact, after most prostate surgeries the amount of ejaculate fluid essentially drops to zero, but orgasms remain just as pleasurable. Also interesting is that an erection is not a requirement for orgasm or ejaculation. Erections are under different nerve control than orgasm, making it possible to still achieve orgasms without erections. Of course, intercourse isn't possible, but if a couple still wants intercourse, there are solutions (see chapter 4).

Many men over sixty have erections more than once a week. However, they may have the urge to ejaculate less often than that. As with women, intercourse without orgasm is still fun and feels good. Penile massage can be satisfying without orgasm. Men who attempt to force themselves toward orgasm every time they have sexual contact can become frustrated and lay the foundation for sexual dysfunction. Men who try too hard to have an orgasm interfere with the relaxation necessary for orgasm to occur.

> *I'm in my late sixties and still enjoy sex. It's changed a little over the years, but it warms me inside and out. One particular thing may seem odd (I never thought I'd hear myself say this!), but sometimes I like intercourse whether or not I have an orgasm. It's the strangest thing, I know, but the old boy just likes the feeling of lots of attention and loves to be massaged, but occasionally doesn't care if that's all there is. It's kind of like enjoying a really great steak, and finding that you really don't need dessert afterward to be perfectly satisfied.*

Age-related changes in both men and women. Orgasmic contractions decrease in number and become farther apart. Although pelvic muscle shrinkage may also reduce contraction strength, orgasms are still enjoyable throughout old age.

All these changes are normal. If you notice that your orgasms are slightly shorter, for example, don't worry that you're losing your sexual abilities or start watching your sexual performance. Focusing too much on function causes anxiety and promotes sexual failure.

Decide that pleasure is the real goal of sex, not orgasm. Sexuality has spiritual and psychological dimensions that are just as valuable. Sex can continue to be satisfying, exciting, and important whether or not you reach orgasm. Lack of orgasm occasionally shouldn't seem like a failure to you. The new goals of sex are delight, satisfaction, and pleasure.

Resolution Phase

Overview. During this phase the physical changes that occurred during arousal and orgasm reverse back to normal as the body relaxes. The resolution phase takes longer if arousal lasted a long time, because entrapment of blood in the pelvic organs is greater. This also happens if arousal occurs without orgasm following.

During resolution men have a "refractory period," a time immediately following orgasm during which they are unable to respond to more stimulation. Even if penile friction continues (which can hurt at this point!), nerve pathways are temporarily resistant to orgasm. Many women are ignorant about this and must be told not to be too sexually demanding after male orgasm because of the refractory period.

Some people feel sleepy after orgasm, while others feel energized. A couple may be at odds if the woman wants to talk, but the man wants to sleep. Each partner must be careful not to misinterpret the postcoital needs of the other. Just because a man immediately drops off to sleep doesn't mean he was only interested in the woman for sex. Likewise, a man shouldn't believe his wife is insensitive just because she wants to go make a sandwich after sex when he wants just to cuddle and doze and recover.

Age-related changes in women. Without adequate lubrication of the vagina and clitoris, a woman will be quite sore after sex. Because friction irritates fragile genital tissues, she may also feel the urge to urinate, particularly after prolonged intercourse. Women approaching and past menopause are especially prone to dryness. One of the first clues that menopause is approaching is soreness after intercourse. Some women misinterpret it as a vaginal infection, but can distinguish by noting the lack of vaginal discharge and monitoring on a calendar when soreness appears and disappears in relation to sexual activity. Women see few other changes in their resolution phase as they age, except some notice that their nipples stay erect longer with or without orgasm.

Age-related changes in men. Lengthening of the refractory period is one of the first signs of aging. At age twenty, a man's refractory period may have been barely perceptible. At age thirty it may last ten minutes, at age forty for thirty minutes, and so forth. One study of male sexuality found that seventy-eight-year-old men had perfectly normal refractory periods lasting five to ten days.

If a man receives sexual stimulation before his refractory period has passed, he *may* be able to achieve an erection but certainly won't have an orgasm. He probably won't have an urge to ejaculate, even with an erection. Some aging couples worry that this signals a sexual dysfunction, but again, this is a normal part of growing older. If a wife wants sex before her husband is able to regain an erection, they must look for other ways to meet her sexual needs or wait. He can provide clitoral stimulation to orgasm through manual stimulation or cunnilingus (mouth-to-clitoris stimulation) or other techniques.

> *Charlie has been just great about this. He says I always did have a stronger sex drive than he did. What we do when I'm in the mood and his body just won't cooperate is that we snuggle up on the couch in front of the TV under a blanket. He picks out his favorite show, and I just let his fingers do the walking. It's actually very romantic. He cares enough to get me through, and I care enough to let him not be bored during it. It's funny, too, how many times he discovers there's a little spark of fire in him after all when he gets turned on by how turned on I've gotten!*

Some women find that trying sex before their husbands are capable of erection or orgasm makes them become anxious, embarrassed, or even angry. These women should masturbate to alleviate their sexual arousal or wait until later, when their husbands are ready.

If an older man loses his erection without having an orgasm, he may have a refractory period anyway. Often this refractory period is shorter than one following an orgasm, though. Once orgasm occurs, erection subsides more quickly with age.

On the positive side, if a man becomes sexually aroused but has no orgasm, he usually doesn't feel the physical discomfort or frustration that a younger man experiences. Since the prostate and seminal vesicles produce less ejaculate fluid and since pelvic organs engorge less with age, there is less physical urgency for ejaculation.

Age-related changes in both men and women. The resolution phase can become more important as couples become more comfortable through the years. Sex evolves away from a race for orgasm and becomes more of a love-oriented interaction. Massage, romance, and companionship give a satisfying holistic feeling of sexual arousal. Growth in intimacy over the years also creates an immense sense of fulfillment and contentment.

THAT AGING PERSON IN THE MIRROR

Even though I don't always recognize that aging person in the mirror, I still cherish her. Her growing list of challenges makes her even more endearing and, for that matter, her husband's make him more precious, too. As we discover new frailties in ourselves and each other, we cling together all the more tightly.

Aging makes us wiser and more comfortable with ourselves. Although our vulnerability to the effects of time increases, we learn how to compensate. Our internal power and external relationships improve. We unveil and appreciate qualities more important than unwrinkled skin and firm muscles and fast orgasms: our love for each other and our families, and our value to God and to society. We are thankful that our spouses age along with us and that we have each other as companions on the journey.

We have the strength to meet the challenges of sexual aging. We know what real sex is and value it. And we're not going to let mere inconveniences or biology or laziness keep us from it.

3

THE SEXUALLY FULFILLED WOMAN

The Book of Proverbs says, "A virtuous woman . . . does not eat the bread of idleness." The world must be full of virtue, since most women are incredibly busy. They keep their households clean, fed, and organized. Many are employed to provide for their families' financial needs; others creatively conserve money as they work at home without pay. They nudge and nurture every family member as wives, mothers, and grandmothers. They achieve work and career goals. In the midst of this busyness, however, too many never become sexually fulfilled as well.

It's not that women don't want sexual fulfillment. Most yearn for the same sexual energy and swift physical response that men have. While female orgasm provides the same intense thrill that male orgasm does, sexual arousal and orgasm are harder to achieve. Female orgasm requires a mixture of concentration, relaxation, and the ability to tune out the environment and worries.

THE UNIQUE COMPONENTS OF FEMALE SEXUALITY

Women Respond to Stimuli Differently Than Men Do

Women are very sensitive to and need touch for sexual arousal more than men do. Merely holding hands, embracing, or dancing closely can provoke vaginal lubrication. By stroking his wife's body and working his way gradually toward her erogenous zones, such as the nipples, earlobes, the inner thighs, and the clitoris, a man can usually bring about vaginal lubrication if she relaxes and desires sex.

Most women are also more reactive to smells than men are. Women like perfume, scented bubble baths, potpourri, incense, and aromatic candles. Likewise, they are more sensitive to unpleasant body odors. Smells are so important that a woman finds it difficult to respond sexually to her husband if he hasn't bathed recently.

Sounds are important, too, both as stimulants and as barriers to sex. Some women believe soft romantic music or rock music with a sensual beat to it is an important background element during lovemaking. Auditory sensitivity can work the opposite way, too, though. Distracting sounds, such as a television on in the room, or even pleasant music, keep many wives from being able to concentrate on sex. Some women think it's helpful to carry on a sexy conversation with their husbands, while others find that talk delays or inhibits sexual response. In general, men function sexually regardless of sounds around them. Women, however, are very sensitive to them and almost always find it's impossible to have sex when they can hear their children or their baby crying.

The old myth that women don't respond to visual stimulation is false. Women do indeed enjoy looking at the male body. The sight of an erect penis can be thrilling, activating fantasies of lusty, boisterous sex. A common female fantasy is to be snared by a man and compelled into sex. (While this may seem like rape, it doesn't reflect a desire to participate in unwanted sex. Rather, the idea that she could be so appealing to a man that he couldn't resist her is very exciting. With real sex, though, a man should exhibit enthusiasm without handling his wife roughly.) Visual images are even more likely to inspire sexual arousal in men. Women require considerably more time of purely visual stimulation to experience the first stage of sexual arousal, such as vaginal lubrication.

Women Take Longer to Reach Orgasm and Have to Concentrate More

The excitement phase of human sexual response is longer for women, especially during partner sex. The buildup toward orgasm also takes some concentration—a foreign concept to most men. Physical stimulation of the penis typically brings about an automatic progression to orgasm, with little effort as long as the contact continues. In fact, the less effort and concentration that men put into reaching orgasm, the more likely they are to achieve it.

Women, however, discover that their thoughts wander easily—even when they want sex. A woman is less likely to get turned on if she lets her mind go blank and doesn't think about anything. Her mind starts to move away from the moment, reminding her that she forgot to write a check for the children's lunch money, didn't get her grandson's birthday card mailed yet, needs to weed the flower beds, has a report due to the boss the day after tomorrow, and a hundred other things. For a woman to achieve orgasm she must clear her mind of distracting thoughts and purposefully pay attention to the sensations her body is feeling, allowing them to build toward orgasm. A paradox of female sexuality is, though, that orgasm takes so much concentrated effort that it can border dangerously close to "performance anxiety." Performance anxiety refers to working so hard to reach orgasm that the mind and the body cannot relax enough neurologically for it to happen.

> *Having an orgasm usually takes at least thirty minutes straight of Ed just rubbing my clitoris. If he slows down or stops to shift positions for just a second, I lose a lot of ground. It's like orgasm is at the top of a hill I'm climbing, but if I get distracted or he stops briefly, I trip and roll halfway back down the hill again.*

Female Anatomy Makes Orgasm More Challenging

Another factor of great importance that makes a woman's ability to reach orgasm more difficult has to do with the size and location of the clitoris. Parents rarely teach little girls about the clitoris. A girl often doesn't discover that she even *has* a clitoris until puberty or beyond. The clitoris is so small and hidden inside the labia that it's impossible for her to see it without a mirror.

The clitoris is more sensitive than the penis, probably because nerve endings are concentrated into a smaller area of tissue. There's a small difference between the amount of pressure that brings pleasure rather than pain, and a minuscule difference between the right location for ecstasy and the wrong location for agony along the short length of the clitoral shaft. While clitoral stimulation is essential for orgasm, it must also be of the right type. Proper clitoral technique is a skill that both the woman and her husband must learn—for example, stimulation of the shaft of the clitoris through the foreskin is pleasurable, whereas direct contact with the tip of the clitoris can be painful—especially during early foreplay.

Women Have Unrealistic Expectations of Men

Women tend to expect men to know intuitively how to make love to a woman. They think that by explaining to men what they want, they are stating the obvious and destroying spontaneity. Female sexual needs and signs of arousal aren't obvious to men, though. It's unfair for women to become angry with their husbands' ineffective techniques or failures to interpret subtle signals if they haven't explicitly stated what they want and need.

For the man whose wife won't verbalize her sexual desires, here are some clues. When she's open to sex, a woman starts by unconsciously flirting, shown by her touching her hair, talking with her head slightly tilted to one side, and shyly looking at you and then quickly looking away. She may try to kiss you and press her body against yours. Generally, touching you above the waist can be a sign of sexual interest or just an affectionate gesture. Touching below the waist is a stronger sexual come-on.

You can gauge how fast to proceed by noting her body language. If she arches her chest toward you, that means she wants you to touch her breasts. If she is rocking her pelvis or separating her knees, she is ready for genital contact. If she keeps shifting her pelvis to move her clitoris farther up or down in relation to your hand, she wants you to touch her clitoris higher or lower on its shaft. If she seems to be backing away from you, she is having pain from too much pressure or not enough lubrication on her clitoris.

If your wife holds very still at some point during clitoral stimulation, she hasn't fallen asleep. She's probably very aroused and is concentrating hard on what you're making her clitoris feel. She's more likely to start moving her pelvis rhythmically during intercourse or as she nears orgasm.

> *For years I couldn't understand why Tanya didn't seem to be more enthusiastic about sex. When I get turned on, my body just starts*

to rock and need motion, and I expected the same from her. One time, though, about fifteen years into our marriage she stopped me right in the middle of lovemaking and said, "Would you please just hold still until I come! You keep distracting me!" Later, I asked her what that was all about, and she said there comes a point when she gets so turned on that she just needs unrelenting, nondistracting rubbing. She said it was kind of like walking a tightrope between the getting turned on part and the last minute before orgasm—fun at the beginning and end, but serious business partway through.

Your wife doesn't want intercourse until her vagina is wet enough, so slide your hand down to her vaginal opening to check for extra moisture. If she doesn't lubricate well anymore even when she is turned on because her estrogen is low, apply artificial lubricant to your penis and her vaginal opening as part of foreplay. If you're not sure if she's ready yet, put your penis near her vagina to see if she starts trying to work it inside. Of course, you should be helping her by this time by thrusting it in little by little. Other clues for readiness for intercourse are that her clitoris has become large and firm, or she is making soft little moaning sounds.

A woman finds it exciting when her husband shows he is comfortable with her body. He can do this by not limiting himself to just the basic techniques of breast massage, rubbing the clitoris, and intercourse. He can add special touches, such as licking the very tips of her nipples or occasionally stroking her labia using several fingers, not just touching her clitoris with the tip of one finger. He slips a finger into her vagina, lifts her hips to meet his penis, and hangs on to her buttocks while he thrusts.

Unfortunately, women who cannot express their needs or may not even know themselves what they need, find sex to be uninspiring. The complexities of female sexuality can cause such frustration that some women give up on orgasms.

Women See the World Differently Than Men Do

Sex means different things to men than to women. Men view sex as a symbol of their adult maleness. Sex has connotations of conquest tied with ego and pride. Sex also provides more physical relief to men through expulsion of accumulated ejaculate fluid.

For women sex is a preciously intimate and emotional gift they give to men. When a woman allows a man to have intercourse with her she is vulnerable to his misuse of her gift. If a man appears insensitive, rejects her, ridicules her, abandons her, or just ignores her after sex, a woman experiences deep personal loss.

It should not be a surprise that men and women differ so greatly in how they respond and view sexuality. Gender differences are apparent from an early age. Unlike what we have heard in recent years, environment is less responsible for many of these differences than we used to think. For example, boys not allowed to have toy guns or watch violence on television still make their own guns out of sticks and fingers and anything else available.

The differences between men and women probably occur as a result of brain imprinting before birth. Under the influence of testosterone for male babies, or the absence of testosterone for female babies, the brain develops in certain ways. Nowhere do differences become so apparent as they do in each gender's view of sex. For men, as long as a woman is reasonably attractive, it's not as important what she looks like as it is how she acts and flaunts her sexuality. Her attitude counts much more than how much makeup she has on or how fancy her hair is.

> *I don't know where I came up with this notion, but I thought that sexiness was perfectly applied makeup, carefully styled hair, perfume, a lacy nighty, and "Isn't It Romantic?" playing in the background. I was always careful to fit that image before dropping any sexual hints to my husband. Always, that is, until the day Jack came home unexpectedly early to find me in a torn T-shirt, wearing no bra, streaked with dirt and sweat, while I was struggling to move some plants into a new flowerbed. My hair was hanging in damp strings and I had no makeup on. I was embarrassed to be caught that way. It was really weird, though, because Jack got this strange gleam in his eyes and starting acting really sultry. Little did I know that I had a man who found the sweaty odor of a woman sexy. All it took was one throaty growl from me in response, and the next thing I knew, he was tearing my clothes off and we were having sex right there in the garage.*

Women feel more inhibited about sexuality and aren't typically like those females on television who flaunt their bodies (unless they are desperately seeking a man). Women have become more assertive about asking for sex and pursuing men than before, but they continue to be vulnerable to shame and hurt when men use sex as a tool for power or selfishness.

Women are touchier about their physical appearances and feel devastated by humor or seemingly harmless remarks about their bodies, especially comments by their husbands. What *do* women want? They want more touching and talking than most men want during sex. Women don't see foreplay as a prelude to something better. It is as valuable as intercourse (although getting turned on and not having an orgasm is very frustrating). Women also like afterplay more than men. Women don't like mechanical sex, where technique is more important than expression. Women want men to touch and stimulate their clitorises and not to quit just when they get turned on enough for intercourse to start.

I've often heard it said that women give sex to get love, and men give love to get sex. There is some truth in this simplistic contrast. Sex has a very strong emotional—even spiritual—component for women. This does *not* mean, of course, that women don't have a sex drive and don't get just as horny as men do sometimes. Even then, though, sex has deeply personal implications for women.

Differences between men and women can create serious problems, such as the inadequate frequency of female orgasm. Many women suffer through marital life not understanding what goes into achieving orgasm. As years pass, others have orgasms less often. Let's consider why orgasms may be absent or infrequent in women's lives and what they can do to become sexually fulfilled.

What Is Anorgasmia?

Anorgasmia means absence of orgasms, a problem in which a woman either has never had an orgasm or for some reason no longer does. In years past the common term for anorgasmia was "frigidity," which implied a woman was sexually aloof, unfeeling, and possessed a cold, unresponsive personality. Frigidity is a slanderous label that causes significant emotional harm and dishonor to a woman. For obvious reasons, it is no longer an acceptable term in sexology.

Anorgasmia is a widespread problem. Every woman at some point in life has difficulty having orgasms. Whether that difficulty turns into a sexual dysfunction depends on how long the difficulty persists, how deeply rooted the difficulty is, and how often she deceives her husband by pretending to be orgasmic.

There is tremendous pressure to succeed at sex, defined as being orgasmic in too many people's minds. Faking orgasms is a symptom of this pressure, which starts as a sporadic way of coping and can turn into a habit. It's astonishing that most women have faked orgasms at least occasionally.

In addition to pressure to be sexually successful, there are other reasons why someone might pretend to be orgasmic. For example, some women would rather fake orgasms than admit to such a personal and potentially embarrassing problem as anorgasmia. For others, it's simple exasperation or inadequate communication.

> *Sometimes I'm just not in the mood for sex, but Frank doesn't take "No" for an answer. I don't mind helping him out, but he thinks we can't quit until I come, too. He just won't stop until he's satisfied that I'm satisfied—meaning I've had an orgasm. Sometimes my clitoris really gets sore after he's worked on me too long, and then there's no way I'm going to be able to get turned on. Once we blew up over it and had a terrible fight. He walked around with hurt feelings for a week. Rather than risk all that again, I've decided it's easier just to fake an orgasm so he'll leave me alone and I can go to sleep in peace.*

Primary Anorgasmia

A woman with primary anorgasmia has never had an orgasm. She isn't sure what an orgasm feels like. Sex therapists like to call women of this type "preorgasmic," supporting the idea that every woman is capable of orgasms.

There are many reasons why a woman may never have had an orgasm. She may lack knowledge about female sexuality and her own anatomy. She may not know how to stimulate her clitoris. Most women who never learn how to bring themselves to orgasm also never have orgasms during partner sex. Women whose religious beliefs condemn masturbation face a special challenge to becoming orgasmic and must depend on their husbands to help them learn. It's unrealistic to expect universal success in such cases, but it certainly is possible if the couple is willing to work together.

> *I grew up in a strict Catholic home where sex was never discussed, but I used to daydream about what sexual ecstasies my future*

husband would give me. When I finally did grow up barely enough to get married, my wedding night was a harsh disappointment. My poor Michael barely knew any more than I did about sex. Sex meant only intercourse and only in the missionary position. To avoid pain I quickly learned to spread some Vaseline on down there before he started, because I never got turned on enough to be wet. Years after Michael's accident and death, I married a wonderful man who introduced me to real lovemaking. I'll never forget the night I had my first orgasm. I was forty-seven years old and a grandmother.

Learning how to properly stimulate your clitoris to orgasm is usually a matter of practice. Start in complete privacy without fear of interruption. Take your time. Note the sensations, location, and types of pressure, friction, and movement that work best. If you think that a book would help, one that has been around for many years but that continues to be a good resource is *For Yourself* by Lonnie Barbach. Once you understand what an orgasm feels like and can achieve orgasms on your own, you can then proceed to teach your husband techniques you would like him to use.

Sexual inhibitions and phobias can also cause primary anorgasmia. These hang-ups come from parental warnings about the "evils" of sex or masturbation. They can also arise from fear of sex, shame, self-consciousness, or embarrassment. Primary anorgasmia rooted in psychological barriers may require professional help, or at least time spent seriously analyzing your background and giving yourself permission to become sexual. Enjoyment of sexuality to the point of orgasm can take a while if your hang-ups are deep seated or shelved in the deep recesses of your brain.

Some women never become orgasmic because they have the attitude that it's their husband's responsibility to "give" them an orgasm. Maybe somebody told them that men are to take the lead in sex. Such women have unrealistic expectations not only of any man's ability to "make" a woman come to orgasm, but also have mistaken ideas about a woman's lack of responsibility. Related to this is when a woman believes her partner should somehow know her thoughts and provide exactly the type of stimulation she needs, but then blames him for her anorgasmia.

Secondary Anorgasmia

In secondary anorgasmia a woman had orgasms in the past but is not currently. Since this problem encompasses most cases of orgasmic dysfunction in older women, we're going to spend some time analyzing its causes and solutions.

WHY ANORGASMIA CAN BECOME A PROBLEM AS YOU GET OLDER, AND WHAT TO DO

Problems with Sexual Technique

For most women, reaching an orgasm is not automatic. The mind is ready and the body is able and sexual desire is strong, but the technique used is inadequate. The first objective should be for your husband to manipulate your clitoris long enough and with the right amount of pressure to neurologically create the buildup needed. Explain to him that stimulation should continue longer than he might expect. Tell him you want him to stroke your inner thighs or French-kiss you or lick your nipples or whatever enhances your arousal.

> *I found it hard to talk about sex with Jim. I had never said such personal things before—even to my girlfriends. I was really surprised that his reaction was surprisingly positive, though, and it got easier the more we discussed it.*

Word your disclosure in a way that conveys you need your husband's help and doesn't come across as criticism of his methods. Most men find it exciting, not crude, for their wives to discuss their sexual needs.

Achieving orgasm with your husband also requires three more elements: relaxation, tenderness, and variety. Relaxation means you feel comfortable and emotionally close to each other. To be relaxed you cannot be angry or upset. You must trust each other, feeling free to touch each other's bodies anywhere and talk without fear of being ridiculed, called kinky, laughed at, or embarrassed later outside the bedroom by each other's remarks. Furthermore, relaxation means that sex is not a race to orgasm (unless you've agreed to have a quickie, which usually means he has an orgasm but you don't).

Second, tenderness connotes caring about each other. It does *not* mean that gentle touching is necessarily always appropriate. Sometimes hot and heavy sex is exhilarating! Instead, tenderness involves asking your husband what he likes, too, teaching him *tactfully* what you want, taking time with each other, being close, enjoying each other's bodies without regard to age or appearance, and devoting attention to one another.

Third, variety is more than sexual spice, it's sexual vitamins. Don't assume that just because your husband responded once to a certain technique, it will work every time. Admittedly, exploring a variety of sexual techniques requires trust because some techniques will fail. Some will end in exasperation or with both of you giggling, which is perfectly fine! It's no big deal if one of you didn't like a particular strategy. Exploring variety itself makes sex more satisfying. On the other hand, don't believe that every encounter must be new and different. That's tiring, too. Herein lies another reason why married sex is better: you don't have to adjust constantly to new techniques or learn to trust a new partner.

Do you need ideas for variety? Change the length of foreplay. A quickie in the living room when the kids are gone is exciting, as are weekends away with hours of foreplay. Speaking of location, foreplay doesn't always have to occur in bed. Start by flirting over dinner, then sit on the couch together to watch television. Sneak a quick grab or pinch in public places or in front of the grandkids. Have sex outside in the dark under the stars on a blanket sometime.

Try oral sex. If you haven't received cunnilingus (stimulation of the clitoris by his tongue and lips) before, ask your husband if he would be willing. Do him a favor by washing your genitals first and trimming your pubic hair if it's very long. Do yourself a favor by abandoning your modesty and inhibitions. Cunnilingus is a delightful technique because it requires no artificial lubrication, focuses on the clitoris, is very sexy, and is more gentle than manual stimulation (tell him not to use his teeth!). It's also sanitary if neither of you has a sexually transmitted disease. (He can give you genital herpes if he has an open cold sore, and you can give him cold sores if you are having a flare-up of genital herpes. Otherwise, normal germs on the genitals are harmless to healthy individuals.)

Vary the types of stimulation. Visually erotic literature (not pornography) is arousing for both men and women and gives inspiration for new techniques. Read a sex manual together. Experiment with sexy clothing and undressing each other. If you usually leave the lights off, turn them on or use soft candlelight.

Add romance by introducing pleasant aromas, starting with a clean body (take a shower together and wash each other!), unless sweat turns you both on. Rub a scented oil or lotion all over him, then ask him to do the same for you. Try visualizing sexual scenes to help you become aroused. Sexual fantasies may involve activities that you might want to act out in reality if given the chance. Don't create a fantasy life in which you have an affair with your husband's best friend or even a movie star. While fantasies are usually arousing because they contain something forbidden, it's best to keep them focused on your husband. Pretend that you're making love in a setting that contains an element of risk of discovery, for example. Recall favorite sexual experiences you've had in the past or scenes from a juicy movie you once saw.

> *My favorite fantasy that never fails to do the trick is really quite simple. I'm embarrassed how tame it is, compared to the stuff I read in my favorite novels. I like to picture myself at work (I'm a high school teacher) judging tryouts for the school play. I'm sitting at a table with a very long tablecloth that reaches to the floor. All of a sudden I feel someone's hands all over my thighs, pulling off my underwear. I can hardly breathe, it feels so good. I peek under the table and see my husband under there with an impish look on his face, knowing how turned on I am and how mortified I would be if anyone caught us.*

When a couple adopts clitoral stimulation as part of sex, they may have to give up traditional intercourse positions that prevent clitoral access. New positions themselves add delightful variety. If you believe the myth that the thrusting movements of intercourse provide enough clitoral stimulation to bring about female orgasm, you're probably wondering why *you* haven't been able to reach orgasm during intercourse. In reality, less than a third of women have orgasms during intercourse. Those who do are able to because the positions they use expose the clitoris to simultaneous manual stimulation. If you still favor a traditional position, let your husband bring you to orgasm before starting intercourse.

Loss of Sexual Desire and "Turnoffs"

The second reason why anorgasmia can become a problem as you age has to do with a diminishing desire for sex or the appearance of something that alters your satisfaction with it. In addition to menopause factors covered in chapter 2, other problems are:

Depression. One widespread cause for lost sexual desire, one we often fail to recognize, is depression. A symptom of depression is lack of interest in sex. If you suspect that you're depressed, you may first want to read *Feeling Good* by David D. Burns; it is a cognitive therapy approach to negative self-talk. However, overcoming depression often requires outside assistance. If you have thoughts about ending your own life, put this book down and call your local suicide hot line this very minute.

Have hope. Depression is very treatable these days. Be advised, though, that some medications used to treat depression, such as Prozac or Elavil, can themselves decrease sex drive. Ask your physician about alternatives.

Stress. As we age, life can become more stressful. While young parents think that nothing could be worse than rearing small children, managing the demands of teenagers or living with the hurt and worry that adult children can bring may cause even deeper anxiety. It's obvious to anyone who has been through more than forty years of life that stress doesn't go away typically. It merely changes form and can intensify as job promotions bring on more responsibility, people depending on us increase in number, our bodies fail us more often, and so forth. Retirement, family tragedies, or entering new career phases bring on worries. Whatever the cause, stress eventually takes its toll on the body, shown by heartburn, headache, anxiety disorder, menstrual irregularities, sleeplessness, heart disease, and changes in appetite. However, stress can also lower testosterone in both men and women, decreasing sex drive in both genders.

Each source of excessive stress requires a different solution. Periodically reassess the pressures you put on yourself and the burdens you accept from others. Decide whether they're worth the problems they cause, particularly if they affect your marriage and sex life.

It wasn't easy for me to consciously decide to make my sexual relationship with my husband a time priority. I've heard for a couple of decades why it's important to take time for myself and that's it's okay to be a little selfish, but this was self-indulgence on a totally new level. It has been so helpful, though. We used to reach a point every so often where we would get progressively more grouchy with each other, and we finally pinpointed the cause. We weren't caring enough about ourselves and our sexual bond. Taking the time to have sex relieves so much tension in our relationship that it's really stupid it took us so long to figure it out.

Substance abuse.   Many substances—even legal ones—dull the senses and affect the libido, such as food. Overeating not only causes weight gain, it also makes our bodies and minds more sluggish and resistant to sexual activity. Alcohol also disrupts arousal and sex drive. Some people start using alcohol just before sex to release their inhibitions or to help them relax. Unfortunately, this can become a habitual pattern. They start to think they *must* have alcohol to function sexually. The longer alcohol consumption continues, the more likely it is that a person will develop a tolerance to it. It starts to take two drinks to accomplish what one used to and escalates to larger amounts over time.

Alcohol not only alters perceptions and decreases judgment, it also sedates and causes so much drowsiness that sleep becomes more attractive than the sexual partner. Alcohol also disrupts sexual arousal by interfering with nerve function. When a woman finds she's unable to become aroused or reach orgasm, she may feel anxiety about her failure—particularly if she doesn't realize alcohol is the cause. As she becomes more anxious and worried about anorgasmia, she may drink more, not knowing she's making the problem worse. Anorgasmia occurs twice as often in female alcoholics as in female nonalcoholics.

It all started with the best of intentions. Larry had early signs of heart disease, so we were working hard to do the right things to reverse it: eating low fat foods, exercising more, taking cholesterol medicine, taking Vitamin E and an aspirin every day, and so forth. I was doing it all, too, because it helped Larry stay on track. One thing we'd heard was that a glass of red wine every day could help reduce heart attacks, so we started having a glass every night at bedtime. I had never been much of a drinker and noticed immediately how much sleepier and warmer it made me. It helped me fall asleep, but gave me lots of trouble when it came time for sex. I just couldn't get up the energy. We solved that problem by having our wine with dinner, but now I get sleepy in the evening while watching TV.

Illegal drugs such as marijuana can also sedate and interfere with sexual desire. Furthermore, they alter the mind's perception of sexual activity. Harder drugs, such as cocaine, completely knock out the sex drive. Eventually the drug high becomes much more important than sex.

Fear, guilt, and inhibitions.   Some women have a deep-seated fear of sex. Perhaps in your background there's a long-kept secret that created fear. Maybe someone planted a seed of anxiety in your mind as a young girl by telling you men are brutes, the penis is too large to fit into the vagina without causing bleeding and pain, or sex is a vile act. Even though you've since learned otherwise, you still may not be able to relax and enjoy sexual intercourse. You may not even want sex.

Maybe your anxiety during sex is based on an experience in which someone really did harm you sexually. Every time you anticipate sex, your insides knot up, you feel a little nauseous, or at least you feel completely disinterested. If you proceed anyway without becoming sexually aroused, intercourse often hurts.

Perhaps your fear is not based on anything so destructive. Some women are just afraid of sex because they're self-conscious or don't like the loss of control that orgasm causes. Maybe your fear of sex is due to pain during intercourse from a vaginal infection, anatomical problem, or something else. Chapter 5 explains what to do when sex hurts.

Some women feel guilt about having sex. They haven't forgiven themselves for an extramarital affair. Maybe they feel they're neglecting their children by taking time for something so hedonistic as sex. Perhaps you have no trouble becoming sexually aroused, but don't make it to orgasm because you feel guilty over how much longer clitoral stimulation takes than penile stimulation.

Karl used to make me so mad. He'd fall asleep right in the middle of turning me on—can you image it?! Boy, did that make me feel boring and selfish or what?! I started thinking about how self-centered I was; I was imposing on his time and generosity for something so selfish. The poor man had been working hard all day, and now I'm forcing him to stay awake past Jay's monologue just so I can have a little whoopee. Then I'd start to get angry. I've got a right to my orgasm, too! It's not fair he can get through in just five minutes, then I have to struggle on for another twenty. How callused can a man be? One night I really let him have it. The poor guy just lay there stunned and stuttering. He said he was sorry about fifty times and would try harder. Of course, that just made me feel like dirt. He did try harder for a few weeks, but would still fall asleep occasionally in spite of it all. I decided there had to be a better way. From then on I wouldn't touch his penis or let him in me (except just enough to make sure he was still turned on), until I had my orgasm first. That works eight times out of ten. The other two times I get myself through or figure "What the heck" and go to sleep.

Factors related to your husband. Difficulties naturally arise when two people of opposite genders with different personalities work together on an issue such as sex. Some challenges that may affect your desire for sex or your ability to reach orgasm are:

1. **A difference in how often you each want sex.** Usually the husband wants sex more often than the wife. His sex drive—indeed, his body's *craving* for orgasmic release—may make him want sex almost daily. His wife, though, needs only one or two orgasms per week. As they age the situation may change: she wants sex once a week and he wants it once a month. The answer isn't necessarily to come to some average between the two extremes, though. They might follow the husband's lead if he wants sex more often, but change their expectations that the wife should have an orgasm every time.

   It's not necessary for a woman to have an orgasm whenever she becomes aroused, unless that's her desire. If you find it hard to become aroused enough to accommodate intercourse comfortably, consider other ways of bringing your husband to orgasm, such as oral sex, or use vaginal lubricant so intercourse is possible without pain.

   When compromising, your attitude is extremely important. You mustn't act as if you are doing your husband a favor or that you're just tolerating his sexual urges. Be gracious with your gift of sex. After all, most women like intercourse whether they have an orgasm or not. If a woman truly loves her husband, she'll find pleasure in seeing him enjoy himself and getting his needs met.

2. **Boredom.** Sometimes one partner thinks the sexual routine has become monotonous while the other finds the routine to be familiar and comfortable. If you're the one who feels bored with your sex life and have communicated that to your husband without getting him to change, or perhaps you've failed to communicate your feelings at all, beware of an insidious buildup of anger against him. The anger that arises from sexual boredom is based on the often faulty belief that your husband doesn't care or is an insensitive clod. If you haven't shared your feelings, though, he can't be blamed. You may discover that your husband would very much like to introduce some variety into your sexual relationship. However, if he does refuse to meet your sexual needs, perhaps the way you ask him is faulty or you both could benefit from marital counseling or sex therapy.

> *I decided if Kirk went through his little routine one more time, I would just scream! For thirty years we made love the same way. Every Saturday night he would lay a towel out at the end of the bed, take off his underwear, play with me until I got turned on (sometimes I even had an orgasm), climb on top, pump until he came, roll off, and go to sleep. Maybe I'm exaggerating a little about how boring it was, but the point is, I needed something different once in a while. One day (a Thursday) I decided I would ambush him and be on top for a change. Even though I wasn't surprising him with leather boots and handcuffs, I was worried he would think I was just as perverted as if I had. Well, he was surprised and a little resistant at first, but he obliged me. The next day he brought flowers home to me and was very affectionate all evening. That night we tried another new position and our sexlife has really flourished since then—all because I finally took the initiative and broke the routine.*

3. **Marital problems.** If your marriage has suffered a blow due to an extramarital affair or other crisis, you'll probably feel dis-

interested in sex for a while. You and your husband must resolve the issue and take active steps to let the relationship heal, assuming you both want to salvage the marriage and seek reconciliation. Even then the respect and trust you lost for your husband will result in a period of sexual difficulty. You may feel repulsed by the idea of having sex with your husband. This doesn't mean you have anorgasmia, only a temporary loss of desire. Often these situations need outside professional help.

4. **Excessive focus on the clitoris.** Some husbands become so well educated about female orgasm that they are overzealous in their manipulation of the clitoris. They focus too much on whether their wives reach orgasm. Behind this problem is a husband who cares about his wife but who may see female orgasm as a reflection of his own skill as a lover. Or he may be using the technique he prefers for his penis, which is more vigorous than what is appropriate for the smaller, more delicate clitoris.

    If your husband attacks your clitoris with too much enthusiasm or acts like he has failed if you don't have an orgasm every time, start by diplomatically teaching him what you need. This kind of revelation often comes across better away from the bedroom when neither of you is feeling particularly amorous. Treat the information you share with him in an objective manner, using a loving and tender approach. Let him know he is helping you and that he hasn't failed as a lover.

5. **He does it his way.** Some husbands believe they must always lead in sex. You can only have sex if it's his idea or if he's the orchestral conductor of all movements. Help him understand that you would also like to lead occasionally, perhaps presenting it in a way that appeals to his secret fantasies of an Amazon who lustily goes after her man.

6. **Pornography.** The occasional use of erotica can be titillating and nurturing to a tired sexual relationship. This type of material or media is not pornography. Rather, pornography deals with sex with children or animals, sadism, masochism, brutality, bondage, humiliation, bizarre imagery, forced sex, and so forth.

    Some men use pornography as a hobby or drug and may

have an addiction to it. A wife who discovers that her husband has this problem may be as hurt as a woman who discovers an extramarital affair. It is a form of mental adultery. She may feel like she has failed to meet his sexual needs and may mistakenly believe she is to blame.

Some husbands share pornography with their wives, hoping it will make them more sexually active and daring. Most wives find it so repulsive that the strategy backfires. They lose their desire for sex altogether.

A pornography addiction is like any other addiction in that it requires professional help to overcome. Spiritual counseling and support groups are beneficial, too.

I'll never forget the day I found that "literature" in Pete's toolbox. I'd always wondered why he had made such a big deal of me leaving his tools alone. What he had in there were several magazines full of naked women missing body parts. I never knew such depravity existed, let alone was published for people to see, let alone that my own husband had a sexual problem with it. I was stunned for days. I didn't say anything to him, and couldn't bear the thought of having sex. I decided he had to be confronted, though, because it was affecting me and our marriage. He was deeply humiliated and even cried—something I had only seen him do a few times. He spilled the whole story, and even seemed to be relieved that he had been caught. Apparently he's had this problem ever since he was in Vietnam. He was just a kid and had never had sex. His buddies set him up with a prostitute who had lost a leg from a land mine. She was nice to him and he was infatuated with her for a while. He got over her, but the sexual link with amputation remained and turned into a habit. I told him he had to get rid of the magazines and give up the fantasies. He agreed, but a few months later I found more. That's when I gave him an ultimatum: Get help or I'm leaving. He got help. It took a long time for me to find him sexually appealing again.

Frequent masturbation.   While masturbation is an important part of a woman's sexual education, there are times when frequent masturbation is a hindrance. The first is when her sex drive is stronger than her husband's—not uncommon as couples age. If your solution is to relieve your own sexual tension, rather than asking your husband to "help you out" without obligating him to intercourse, be careful you don't masturbate so frequently that when he does want sex, you're no longer in the mood. While it does relieve sexual tension by decreasing a woman's libido, *frequent masturbation lengthens the amount of foreplay needed for orgasm during partner sex*. Limit the frequency of masturbation to receive the reward of a more intense and urgent sexual experience when you as a couple share it.

Masturbation also provides a quicker, more intense orgasm because you know the right pressure and stimulation to give your own clitoris at every step of buildup to orgasm. Building a dependence on the most direct route to orgasm also becomes a problem for women who masturbate using a vibrator, a shower massager, or other method that unnecessarily provides a very intense type of stimulation. Manual stimulation by a partner cannot physiologically compete. The subtle strokes and meanderings of clitoral stimulation provided by a partner, which would be more than adequate for a woman whose clitoris does not get frequent intense stimulation, are insufficient for the woman accustomed to much more powerful clitoral massage. This in no way implies that orgasms from masturbation feel better than those your husband gives. The opposite is true. An orgasm given by your husband is like satisfying hunger with a gourmet meal instead of settling for the soda crackers of masturbation.

Changes in Health That Make Orgasms More Difficult

Fatigue.   You may be too weary at the end of the day for sex because of stress, poor physical fitness, or overwork. More serious problems that also cause fatigue include illnesses or deteriorating physical conditions. Regardless of why you're tired, when it's time to have sex, you'll be tempted to think it's not worth the effort.

What are the solutions? First, analyze your lifestyle for obligations that unnecessarily use up your energy. Switch sex to the morning or the afternoon. Most couples find that this gives them the stamina needed for sex and that they feel refreshed afterward, particularly if they take time for a short nap following lovemaking.

Avoid alcohol for three hours before sex because it is a sedative and a relaxant. The same is true of large meals. Eating too much causes drowsiness.

Consider the sexual techniques you use. If you stay with traditional forms of intercourse, such as the man-on-top (missionary) position, you'll find they become more difficult as your husband ages because of the weight he must bear to avoid putting too much pressure on your chest. Other positions work better to conserve energy. For example, the female superior method, in which a man lies on his back and the woman straddles him, allows her to bear weight on her knees and also makes the clitoris more accessible.

In another position the woman is on her knees with her bottom up and her head down on a pillow; her husband kneels behind her. A variation of the rear approach is even more relaxing, in which both partners lie on their sides with the woman's back to her husband's chest, lying like spoons nested in a drawer. To get the penis into the vagina using this position, the woman needs to angle her back away from her husband's chest.

Another relaxing position has the husband lie on his side facing his wife, and she lies on her back. By putting her leg nearest him over his hip or bringing her knee up, she can expose her vaginal opening for intercourse. Neither partner has to bear any weight, and the husband can maneuver to reach her clitoris. Again, it helps to angle the upper bodies away from each other. Experiment to find other positions you like even better that conserve your strength.

Headaches. We've all heard the old joke about the wife who says, "Not tonight, dear. I have a headache." Sometimes, though, headaches are a real problem. The standard solution is to treat the headache before trying to have sex. Take a pain reliever; ask your husband to massage your neck and back to relax tense muscles; or take a long, warm bath before bedtime. If you are among the few people who get headaches during or after orgasm, that is an entirely different matter possibly related to increased blood pressure or elevated pressure inside your head brought on by orgasm. In that case, see your physician, but don't let orgasm headaches make you leery of sex. They're not dangerous, but may be a symptom of an underlying problem worth investigating.

Leaking urine. Leaking urine during orgasm (and at other times) is a problem for millions of women as young as their forties. Pelvic muscles and ligaments weaken from age and having babies, causing the bladder and the uterus to sag. Sphincter muscles controlling urine flow lose tone. Untreated urinary tract infections leave the bladder weakened and prone to urine retention even though we think we've expelled every drop.

Make an appointment with your family doctor or gynecologist to check for an infection. Ask whether you should get your bladder or uterus surgically "pinned back up" where it belongs. Some medications can reduce urine leakage, too. While you wait for your appointment, do Kegel exercises several times a day. (Rapidly squeeze and release the muscles that start and stop your urine flow, as many times as you can. Also, pretend your vagina is a well with a bucket in it. Pull the bucket up to the top of the well as slowly as you can and hold it there.) For two hours before sex, limit the fluids you drink, then empty your bladder completely before starting. If all else fails, put a thick towel under you to soak up any leakage, and keep a sense of humor about it. If your husband asks, assure him that normal urine is sterile. Sex involves so much moisture anyway, he probably won't even notice if you don't mention it. Of course, maintain good hygiene to avoid urine odor, and wear an absorbent pad as needed during your daily routines.

> I started leaking urine in my early fifties whenever I sneezed. My sister had the same problem, so I wasn't all that surprised. That didn't make it any less embarrassing, though. I learned to cope with it and to wear a sanitary napkin (and I had been so happy to quit buying those things after menopause!). It wasn't so bad, though, except during sex. Did you ever try to relax and have an orgasm while keeping your urine muscles tight enough not to leak? It's almost impossible. I finally decided I couldn't let it rule my life—if I leaked, I leaked. The funny thing is, Howard never mentioned it, and I really don't think he even knows. I do stop drinking after dinner and try to pee before sex, though, which help quite a bit.

Nerve degeneration or damage.   Whenever a disease or physically traumatic event affects the nerve tracts into and inside the pelvis, there is risk that the genital organs (especially the clitoris and the labia) might become less sensitive to touch or even numb. If you have diabetes, it may be due to progressive nerve degeneration. This can also be a symptom that you have diabetes but don't know it. If you've had pelvic or rectal surgery, you may have damage both to nerves that carry signals for sensation of touch as well as nerves that cause engorgement. Spinal cord injury and strokes cause severe nerve problems related to orgasm. Nerve degeneration or damage is not reversible. For information on how to adjust sexually, see other sections in this book addressing each type of problem.

Loss of androgens.   Androgens, such as testosterone, are male hormones largely responsible for the sex drive in both men and women. The female body makes androgens in the ovaries and the adrenal glands. Any condition (such as adrenal insufficiency) that affects these organs or having them removed surgically results in testosterone deficiency. With the loss of sex drive, it becomes more difficult to reach orgasm. For more advice on how to deal with low testosterone affecting the female sex drive, see chapter 6.

Kidney disease.   Kidney disorders affect many body systems. Problems include difficulty regulating blood pressure, toxin buildup in the blood, less efficient clearing of certain medications from the body, weakness, and so forth. Since kidney disease can reduce stamina, there may be less energy available for sex. Chronic problems with the kidneys cause more sexual problems for men than for women. Women may note, though, that if the disease progresses to the point where kidney dialysis becomes necessary, hyperprolactinemia (one of the typical changes in hormones that results) often causes cessation of menstrual periods and loss of libido. High blood pressure medicines may decrease genital engorgement during sexual arousal. A woman should explore the options of alternative treatments and medications with her physician as part of her effort to retain her sexual interest and orgasmic ability.

Spectatoring

"Spectatoring" is a term sex therapists use to describe a problem in which some people are so concerned about sexual performance that they start watching themselves and their sexual progress. This can reach a point where they become unable to function sexually. Pressure to "perform" can come from within yourself, or it can come from your husband. Either of you may expect that you should have an orgasm during most (if not every) sexual encounter, but this isn't realistic. We all occasionally find it difficult to become aroused. We might be too tired one night or have too much on our minds. We may have had too much to drink or not be in the mood. We may simply not know why our genitals don't seem to be working.

It's those times when we don't know why we are having trouble performing that we are at greater risk for self-doubts about our sexuality. When we don't become aroused or have an orgasm, the next time we have sex we're likely to watch to see if the problem happens again. We try extra hard to get turned on or to have an orgasm just to prove to ourselves or our spouses that everything is fine.

This is where we can fall into a paradoxical trap, though. The body operates in such a way that the harder we try to have an orgasm, the less likely it is to happen. All our lives we've heard that we can accomplish anything we want to if only we want it badly enough and try hard enough. That simply isn't true when it comes to success at having orgasms. For the human to become sufficiently aroused to reach a sexual climax, our nervous systems have to be relaxed; otherwise, certain parts of them cannot function when we are feeling tension or anxiety. Perhaps you have heard of the "fight or flight" reaction, a nervous system mechanism in which our bodies become more tense and watchful when we worry or have fears. The nerve pathways responsible for sexual arousal cannot function when we are in the "fight or flight" mode.

As we are playing the spectator, while simultaneously trying to be a player at the game of sex, we more often than not fail again. This makes us even more anxious and worried. The next time we try to have sex, we are more concerned, so we watch ourselves more closely to analyze the problem and put out even more effort to reach orgasm.

> *I felt such shame and embarrassment over my sexual failures. My husband even felt he was somehow responsible and started to see himself as a failure, too. As more failures piled up, we'd try even harder and would fail again, and would try harder yet and fail, and would try very hard and fail yet again. It began to affect our relationship and my feelings about myself.*

If you've developed this sexual dysfunction and it has a strong grip on your self-confidence, get professional help from a certified sex therapist. If this is an occasional problem or has only recently begun to crop up, the following information will guide you through some of the more common techniques sex therapists use to bring couples back into a satisfying sex life complete with orgasms.

First, stop having orgasms. Just take a vacation from sex for a while. Tell your husband about the vicious circle that you have fallen into and how frustrated you've become. Ask him to help you rediscover the pleasure of sex. Explain the need to stop having intercourse, assuring him that it is only temporary. Abstain from any sexual contact for at least two or three days and for as long as a week before starting the exercises. This accomplishes two things: (1) it takes the pressure off you to "perform" so that you can let yourself relax mentally and emotionally, and (2) it will help increase sexual desire as your body rebuilds some sexual tension.

When you feel ready, set up an appointment with your husband for a time alone when you know there will be no distractions or interruptions. During this session you will remain clothed and practice "sensate focusing." Sensate focusing helps you to become aware again of the sensual nature of touch outside of the sexual context. It's a relaxing way of receiving and giving touch that will eventually carry over to genital contact. For now, though, limit sensate focusing to exploration of each other's hands and faces. Take turns touching these body parts fully, noticing every texture, muscle, and line. Give each other pleasure by massaging these body parts gently. Be sure you take turns. Do not explore each other simultaneously. It's important to learn to give pleasure while fully concentrating on your husband's reactions and needs, and then to be passive and receive pleasure, letting yourself be totally relaxed and selfish as you enjoy his touch. Take your time. This session should last at least thirty minutes. Later hold hands as you watch television, sit in church, or go for a walk.

Your next appointment together must again be alone and un-interrupted. This time you will proceed through the same exploratory exercise, only now you will remove only enough clothes to give each other back rubs and foot rubs. Use the same methods, and remember that the purpose is to focus on the sensation of both giving and receiving. Do not let this progress on to intercourse, or even any type of sexual contact *yet*.

"Nondemand pleasuring" may seem peculiar and unnatural if you and your husband have strayed away from nonsexual physical contact over the years. However, it's an important step in your growth and sexual adjustment. Remember, orgasm is not the goal of physical contact, or even of sex itself. We must shift our minds away from constantly feeling pressured to reach orgasm and remember that the true goal of sexuality is pleasure.

> *Nondemand pleasuring opened up a new dimension of delight to Chet and me. It started out as a way for us to get reacquainted with the real purpose of lovemaking. It did do that, but we were surprised at how glorious we felt after giving each other an all-over body massage. Now when Chet comes home frazzled and steamed after work, I get out the baby oil and work him over as long as my strength holds out. He does the same for me, too. We don't always have sex afterward, but we feel marvelous! It's incredible how good a total body massage feels. It has brought us closer and has been a real blessing for reducing stress and making us feel loved. It is also makes our skin tingle and warms our muscles. It's a great workout!*

The next time you and your husband set up an appointment alone, you can completely undress and proceed to the next level. Start with a back rub. Then ask him to sit back against the headboard. He then should open his legs wide so you can sit with your back against his chest. Put your head on his shoulder and relax. (If this position is difficult for you, any other you'd prefer will also work as long as you are both comfortable.) Tell him step by step what you want for him to do to give you pleasure—short of genital contact. For example, ask him to kiss your ear and your neck, stroke your breasts, roll your nipples gently between his fingers, rub your tummy, massage your thighs, and so forth. Express your happiness as he succeeds, telling him how good it feels. If this seems like an odd thing for you to do, just purr with pleasure or smile. Try guiding his hands, particularly to show him the type of pressure or movement you like best. Trade places and do the same for him.

The next session repeats the last session, adding genital massage. The best position for this is for him to sit against the headboard with you flat on your back facing him, resting your thighs over his legs. This gives him easy access to your genitals. Trade places when it's his turn. Take turns receiving genital caresses and massage, guiding and explaining what feels best as you proceed. Many couples find this particular session to be so sexually arousing that they have great difficulty resisting the urge to copu-late. You will, of course, decide for yourselves whether to proceed to intercourse or orgasm, but try to wait. Moving toward orgasm the first time your husband touches your genitals is too reminis-cent of your old pattern. Focus purely on the pleasure, but don't have an orgasm. If your husband is going crazy by now, bring him to orgasm *without intercourse.*

Don't have more than one session per day. After as many ses-sions as you want (usually a couple of sessions of genital massage without orgasm are adequate), give yourself permission to have an orgasm *if it happens without effort.* Keep your thoughts fo-cused only on how good his touch feels. Do not plan to have an orgasm. If one happens by accident, that's great and wonderful. Congratulate yourself on breaking out of your vicious circle. How-ever, orgasm is no longer your goal. Relieve yourself of that bur-den, remembering that pleasure is now your new goal.

Thereafter, if you feel sufficiently aroused and have adequate vaginal lubrication and your husband wants intercourse, then certainly give him that gift. You are under no obligation, however, to come to orgasm. What is more important is that you and your husband are sharing an intimate experience that brings great happiness and leaves you both feeling satisfied and loved. Most women by far, though, will resume having orgasms as a wonder-ful bonus to this newfound sexual goal of pleasure for its own sake.

EATING THE BREAD OF IDLENESS

A virtuous woman is indeed one who shuns idleness, even when it comes to sexuality. You are responsible for proactively moving toward your own sexual happiness. It won't come by just sloth-fully hoping for it. It's your duty as a marital partner to know yourself and to teach your husband how to know you more fully. It's a terrible waste—if not a sin—for you to give up. Don't tell yourself that sex isn't that important anymore or that you're too old for sex anyway. You still have so much sexual potential and pleasure to give and to get. If you idly let that potential die, you risk living in a sad and lonely marriage. Get professional help if the suggestions offered here can carry you so only far. Have courage and know that the rewards are sweet. You will feel better physically. You will like yourself more. Your husband will honor you for doing it.

4

PRESERVING MALE
SEXUAL FUNCTION

While male sexuality doesn't include the complexities of a cycling hormonal system and the discomforts of its eventual shutdown as the sexuality of women does, men are more psychologically vulnerable and neurologically complicated than women sexually. Male arousal, erection, orgasm, and ejaculation are not the straightforward mechanisms most women think.

THE UNIQUE COMPONENTS OF MALE SEXUALITY

Before we can understand erectile problems, we need to understand how men view sex and themselves as sexual beings. How are men unlike women?

Men Perceive Sex Differently Than Women Do

Sex is instinctive for men, but not intuitive. While a husband usually cares deeply about his wife's sexual happiness, he's probably not as good a mind reader as she expects him to be. A wife must tell or show her husband what to do for her, but not because he is stupid or uncaring. Instruction is necessary because the brains of the two genders differ in how they function (see "Women Have Unrealistic Expectations of Men" in chapter 3).

Women also misinterpret the male sexual instinct by expecting men to have the same romantic thoughts that they do during sex. When men are in the throes of passion they totally focus on the sensations in their genitals. Their minds are in neutral, but their bodies are accelerating. This explains why men don't fantasize or romanticize as much as women do during sex because, after all, they *already are* having sex. Men don't understand why at that point a fantasy would be necessary.

On the other hand, when a woman opens her mouth in the middle of foreplay or intercourse to ask, "What are you thinking about?," she wants to hear her husband's sexual thoughts so she can enjoy them, too. Or perhaps she asks because she's worried foreplay is having to last so long to meet her needs that he's becoming bored. Men usually reply to this question, "Nothing." For a woman, whose mind typically races during sex, this answer is unbelievable. She imagines, "He must be thinking something really awful about me or he's having a fantasy so bizarre he's afraid I'll think he's a pervert if he tells me." Out of burning curiosity she pressures him some more to tell her. Men don't know how to respond when a woman asks, "What are you thinking about?" during sex because they truly are not thinking, they are feeling and experiencing and riding the surge toward orgasm.

Another difference is that the average man likes a woman to behave seductively, by giving that "come hither" look, moving with exaggerated hip action, pressing her breasts against him, and generally acting provocative. Women tend to show interest in sex instead by behaving romantically, wearing feminine clothes and perfume, playing soft music, kissing, lighting candles, and other less blatantly erotic moves. A woman who adjusts her sexual style to include behaviors her husband is more likely to respond to will be more successful at interesting him in sex. The opposite is true, too. If he can incorporate some romance into his approach, she'll respond better.

I found it incredibly hard to fulfill my husband's sexual fantasies. They weren't kinky or anything, but even his simple request that I do a striptease for him went against everything my mother taught me about how a lady behaves. I did try—really!—but always soon fell into embarrassed giggles. My solution was to let him watch strippers on tape while I was right there to take advantage of the effect it had on him. I know most women put down "bimbos" for how they strut and seduce men, but deep down we're jealous and wish we had that same power to turn men on, too.

Women find it especially odd that men don't necessarily need to have a personal relationship or to feel love to become turned on by a woman. Male response is more automatic, rapid, and triggered merely by the physical attractiveness of a woman. They do, of course, still have control over their actions in spite of the reflexive nature of their "sexual activation switch." They are not responsible, though, for what tempts them and for their automatic sexual reflexes.

Men feel at their most masculine during sex. Without his sexual capacity a man feels as if he is "half a man," because sex is the physical manifestation of being male. Intercourse and oral sex are both important hallmarks of male sexuality. Men sometimes find long foreplay to be frustrating. While long, slow lovemaking is terrific, they think quickies are even better.

Men and women also differ in terms of sex drive strength. The male libido builds to an intensive peak during the late teens and early twenties and is stronger than the sexual peak a woman reaches in her thirties or forties. It's interesting to compare studies on one indicator of the sex drive, that of how often a person has sexual thoughts. Amazing to women is that at the peak of male sex drive, men think about sex several times an hour, whereas a woman at her peak has a sexual thought once or twice a day. Sex is such an overwhelming urge to young men that it almost becomes an obsession. As men age the obsession subsides, but it remains a strong interest for the rest of their lives, even into their eighties and nineties.

During their forties men find that sex becomes more than a physical act, that it has evolved into an important way to communicate intimacy and love to their wives. Because of this dual component to male sexuality, decreasing strength of the sex drive over the years has more to do with a reduction in the physical need for orgasm, not necessarily a decline in desire, which remains quite strong throughout life.

Men Fear Sexual Failure More Than Women Do

When young, a man's anxieties center more on his inability to control the timing of erections and the speed of orgasms. Erections happen at any time for seemingly no apparent reason, bringing about some of life's most embarrassing moments. Orgasms come so quickly that he and his partner are surprised they are over already.

At about ages forty to fifty the anxiety changes to concerns about not getting an erection at all or being put down because of the inability to "perform." Although some men fake orgasm during intercourse, a man cannot fake erections. To restore erections, many are willing to inject drugs into their penises; spend large amounts of money on drugs, devices, herbs, and potions; or have surgery for penile enlargement or implantation of mechanical prostheses into their penises.

> When I began having trouble getting my penis to cooperate, I was really scared. I knew a couple of guys whose sex lives were totally dead and it seemed like all their energy had died, too. I just panicked. I didn't know what to do. I certainly didn't want anyone to know about it, especially Patty. She kept coming on to me and dropping clues and strutting her stuff, but I just pretended I was too tired or mad. I know she was hurt and confused, especially after this went on for several weeks. She started thinking I didn't love her anymore. I tried to convince her that there wasn't anything wrong with her and that I still loved her, that I just wasn't interested in sex anymore. It seemed to be easier to let her think that than admit I still craved her body but I couldn't get my penis to work. I just couldn't face the humiliation.

Men Have Different Concerns about Their Sexual Appearance

While women are preoccupied with their personal appearance and are extremely self-conscious about their bodies, men worry more about how their genitals look. "Is my penis big enough? Are my balls too hairy? Should I get circumcised? Should I have my circumcision reversed? Does my penis have too much of a bend or an angle to it? Should I have plastic surgery to make my circumcision look less ragged?" and so forth.

Once and for all let me, as a woman, as a professional who has seen many naked men in the line of duty, and as a sexologist, settle this matter. Any size of penis is wonderful and satisfying and big enough and awesome to a woman. Anything so much bigger than the clitoris that enlarges so dramatically in response to her attentions is impressive. Any size of penis fits any size of vagina, because the vagina is elastic. The male genitalia are not ugly, but magnificent to a woman—whether they're smooth or hairy, ragged or trimmed, circumcised or uncircumcised (some women are more accustomed to seeing a circumcised penis, but that doesn't mean uncircumcised penises aren't sexy, too), or any other variation possible. What's thrilling and important is the fact that they are *so male*.

The more rugged and hairy a man's genitals are, the more sexually excited a woman may feel because such attributes are typically more masculine than feminine. The smoother and less flawed a man's genitals are, the more sexually excited a woman may feel because those features appeal to her sense of aesthetics. Am I being contradictory? No, because when a woman loves her husband, his genitals are the ones she prefers and finds thrilling, regardless of what they look like. As long as a man keeps himself clean, tends to the normal upkeep of his body, and avoids emitting unpleasant odors and sounds, that's enough to satisfy most women.

Men Feel More Responsibility for the Sexual Happiness of Both Partners

Sometimes it seems to men that they do all the work. They feel pressure to be always ready for sex, to get erect quickly, stay erect, provide their wives with just the right foreplay, bring them to orgasm, and to do it often. Most men would rather by far have wives who are demonstrative, who act sexy *around them*, and who ask for what they need.

Sometimes men prefer masturbation because it is so quick and simple, a fast pressure release valve without concern for someone else's happiness. It's helpful, too, because men can feel bombarded by sexual stimuli everywhere they look (on television, in ads, by women at work, and so forth). Occasionally an older man uses masturbation when he hasn't ejaculated for a month or so, since he no longer has "wet dreams." He knows from experience that if he doesn't relieve fluid pressure building in his prostate, the next time he ejaculates during sex with his wife he'll have pain.

Men need their wives to admire and appreciate them. They need their wives to tell them what good lovers they are and how grand their penises are (yes, even how *big* their penises are—although any erect penis looks huge to a woman). A wife's admiration will go a long way toward keeping a husband faithful if he hits midlife wondering whether he is still attractive sexually.

Men Need a Firmer Touch and More Variety Than Women Do

By age fifty most men need direct physical stimulation of the penis to reach full erection. Whatever their age, men basically want firm stroking of the penis along the entire shaft, particularly around the "head." They like manual stimulation, oral sex (sucking and licking), and intercourse. Each technique serves a different purpose.

> *Alice could never understand why I kept after her to give me fellatio [stimulation of the penis by her mouth]. She said that it just didn't seem "necessary" to her, and she thought it was unsanitary. I'm always careful to be clean, though. I guess I like it because it gives a whole different sensation than intercourse. I like being able to relax and let a woman give me that much attention. I sometimes get tired of long foreplay to get her through, so why can't she oblige me sometimes? Besides, it's great to enjoy my own private sex show. It's my secret fantasy to watch Alice work on me. It would be such a sexy thing for her to do. You'd think she'd be glad to do it for me, because I sure wouldn't let any other woman try it!*

Women who don't like fellatio usually say it's because it seems repulsive to put something in the mouth from which urine comes. They also complain that fellatio gags them, makes their jaws hurt, or they dislike having semen in their mouths. Perhaps they need an attitude adjustment or should use different methods. Here are the facts:

- The washed penis doesn't taste like urine.
- Fellatio doesn't have to be so deep or constant that it gags or makes the jaws ache. She can vary her technique or position as needed to adjust.
- Semen doesn't feel different than lukewarm cream or taste any stronger than vanilla pudding.
- Swallowing semen is optional.
- The genitals are no more "germy" than the mouth if both partners are free of sexually transmitted diseases.

If a woman can overcome her squeamishness about fellatio, she should honor her husband's request. She can try to see it as a privilege and a sign of her husband's trust in her to put himself into such a vulnerable position.

Men like the feel of bare female skin along their bodies. They like the view of a partially naked woman who strips just for them. They like hip action and seductive behavior. Some men like their nipples touched and kissed, while others don't. Most men enjoy having the scrotum and testes gently squeezed and lightly massaged. If the woman can reach the perineum (the area behind the scrotum in front of the anus), she may find that her husband likes having this erogenous zone stroked, too.

Some men welcome anal stimulation; many are repulsed by it. Anal and rectal sexual techniques should never be forced onto anyone. They do carry health risks. Wash anything that touches the anus or goes into the rectum before it touches any other body part. Microbes from the anal area can cause serious infection if transferred to the urinary tract, the vagina, the eyes, and so forth. If using a latex glove over a finger or a condom over the penis, remove it carefully and discard it immediately. Insertion of anything into the rectum is dangerous if not done slowly and with plenty of lubricant. Fragile tissues lining the rectum are easily perforated, risking a life-threatening abdominal infection.

Immediately after orgasm men tend to want all movement to stop immediately, because the refractory period following male orgasm renders them incapable of further arousal for a while and makes continued stimulation painful. Women often appreciate gentle clitoral massage after orgasm that gradually subsides or may even build into another orgasm. As men age, they need longer and more direct penile stimulation for full erection. Older men appreciate less strenuous routes to orgasm, particularly positions and techniques that don't require as much thrusting work.

WHAT IS ERECTILE DYSFUNCTION?

In response to sexual stimulation, the penis expands in length and thickness, becoming fuller and stiffer due to the engorgement of three spongy tissues within its shaft. The two "corpora cavernosa" run parallel along the top, and the corpus spongiosum runs the length of the penis underneath. A man becomes sexually aroused in two possible ways: (1) his brain senses sexual input, or (2) reflex nerve pathways in his spinal cord sense penile stimulation. Penile nerves direct the arteries to expand, allowing blood to flow into the penis more rapidly. When the spongy bodies fill with blood, they put pressure on the veins through which blood drains out of the penis, restricting the speed at which blood can exit.

The nerves that promote erection are not the same ones that bring about orgasm. In fact, it's possible for a man to have an orgasm without an erection. Ejaculation, the expulsion of semen during orgasm, cannot occur without orgasm, though. However, orgasm can occur without ejaculation, as in men who've had their prostates removed and in other cases.

Erectile dysfunction is the inability to achieve an erection or to maintain it until orgasm. The layperson tends to continue calling this problem "impotence," as well as many health care professionals who try to use a term the public recognizes. However, just as the term "frigidity" carries negative connotations, so does the word "impotence." Impotence means a man has lost his erectile ability, but implies he has lost power as a masculine being as well. Therefore, sex therapists prefer the term "erectile dysfunction" or "erectile failure" over "impotence."

> *I've always hated that word—impotence. For some reason it makes me angry. I take it very personally when any man is said to have "impotence," as if it were a slam against all men. I can't explain it. It's just that that word hits me in the gut as surely as if someone had said, "You're not a man," and slugged his fist into me. It castrates male dignity and strength.*

The slowing of arousal and decreasing firmness of erections with normal aging do not constitute an erectile problem. Too many uninformed men assume that something is wrong when they start needing longer foreplay and direct stimulation of the penis to reach a full enough erection to accomplish intercourse. Too many believe that softer erections and prolonged refractory periods signal the beginning of the end of their sexual years. However, these are normal and expected changes that have nothing to do with erectile dysfunction. A man's erectile ability can last to the end of his days (sometimes with medical help).

Another phenomenon some men mistake for an erection problem is that they have trouble getting another erection after losing one without orgasming first. This, too, is normal. By age seventy or so, the refractory period lasts several hours or even days regardless of whether there was an orgasm. (See chapter 2 for more information.)

Psychological versus Physical Erection Problems

Sexologists used to believe that erectile problems were almost always caused by something psychological—that a man's difficulty with erection had more to do with what was going on in his head than what was happening between his legs. We now know that most men who have erection dysfunction have something physically wrong, particularly if they are over forty years old when the problem starts. We're going to examine both the psychological and the physical causes of erectile failure, but first it may help to know some of the ways to tell them apart.

Psychologically induced erectile dysfunction tends to evolve from situations in which some mental or environmental or relationship factor causes difficulty becoming aroused during one or a series of sexual episodes. The man may not consciously recall the particular episode or episodes in question. He will, though, recognize the anxiety that the apparently sudden failure had on his sexual confidence. This rather abrupt onset is an important marker because when a physical problem causes erectile dysfunction, it tends to creep up gradually over months and years. A man with diabetes can look back and say, for example, "Six months ago I was having erections 90 percent of the time when I wanted to, but now I'm lucky if it's 50 percent of the time." A man whose problems are probably psychological in origin recalls, "It practically happened overnight. I was doing fine and then all of a sudden it seemed as though I couldn't have an erection to save my life."

Another way to distinguish between whether an erectile problem is psychological or physical in origin is to note whether erections still occur at times other than during sex. For example, many men have a partial or full erection upon waking in the morning when their bladders are full. If that continues, this is a clue the problem may be psychological. If a man continues to get an erection while masturbating or while with one woman and not another, again this points to a psychological problem.

If you're having erection problems, start by getting a thorough physical examination, being sure to mention that erections are more difficult to obtain than before. If your physician doesn't know how to do a sexual exam, see a residency-trained, board-certified family physician, internist, or urologist who does. Avoid "impotency clinics" at this stage of the investigation. Too often the personnel at these clinics prescribe their favorite drugs and operations without identifying and correcting the underlying cause or providing sex therapy sometimes needed.

The qualified physician will look for evidence of a physical reason for your erectile difficulty. He or she will inspect and feel your scrotum and perineum and possibly use an electronic device to check for normal sensitivity to pressure. If the testes have less sensation and don't register pain as quickly, a disease process may have damaged nerves that transmit messages of arousal into an erection. You'll also have a rectal exam and your prostate evaluated for enlargement, tumors, or infection.

Your physician will check the pulse and blood pressure in your penis to compare with other parts of your body to see how well blood flows into your penis. Since most men have three to five erections every night during sleep, you may undergo a test for two or three nights for "nocturnal tumescence." For this, your penis wears a pressure-sensitive device that monitors for erections. Perhaps you've heard of the "postage-stamp test," in which a man wears a loop of stamps sealed into a circle around his penis while he sleeps. If the loop pops open by the next morning, supposedly he's had an erection during the night. This test is unreliable, though, because movement can dislodge the seals. Devices to monitor penile expansion during sleep are more dependable.

Your physician will also measure your testes. Testicular shrinkage is usually accompanied by decreased testosterone production, causing loss of sex drive and erectile ability. Blood tests for the following are important, too: thyroid hormone, prolactin, luteinizing hormone (LH), follicle-stimulating hormone (FSH), cholesterol, estrogen, blood sugar (glucose), and testosterone. It may help to undergo arteriography, blood vessel studies that reveal possible pelvic or penile artery blockage. Unfortunately, as you age you may not only build up cholesterol and plaque in the arteries to your heart and brain, but also to your penis.

What's important here is not to resort to any erectile treatment without first investigating your physical health. Be skeptical of anyone who sells an "impotence cure" without conducting a complete examination. No physician should prescribe any treatment without checking for diabetes, a tumor on your spinal cord, artery disease, or other serious problems described.

> *My best friend went to one of these "men's health centers" for his impotence. A doctor gave him a quick checkup, which included no lab work, and talked him into learning how to give himself injections to get erections. No other options were discussed. Some assistant did the actual teaching. He got charged two thousand dollars by the time it was over, none of which his insurance covered. He hated doing the injections and gave it up not long after. A few months later his family doctor found out my friend had diabetes, which explained a lot about his impotence.*

WHY ERECTIONS CAN BECOME A PROBLEM AS YOU AGE, AND WHAT TO DO

Even if a definitive physical cause explains an erectile problem, difficulty with function can lead to lost sexual confidence and lost self-esteem.

> *In my case it was a little like arguing, "Which came first, the chicken or the egg?" I was having headaches and finally went to see my doctor. He diagnosed high blood pressure. Part of my treatment included taking medicine. He didn't say anything about side effects, so when I became impotent it never occurred to me that it might be the prescription I was taking. I just figured my body was finally falling apart. I had recently turned fifty and decided I must be over the hill sexually, too. Margaret insisted I mention it to my doctor, though. Then he told me it could be the medicine and switched me to something else. I'd already bought into the idea that my sex life was over, however. I was so dejected that even when I was physically able to have sex again, it took me several weeks to believe in myself enough to get to where I could have intercourse.*

Psychological Causes of Erectile Dysfunction

Men walk a delicate balance between sexual confidence and shame. Many circumstances that cause loss of self-assuredness seep into sexual areas as well. Let's examine some causes of psychologically induced erectile difficulties.

Depression and stress.   Depression in men often intertwines with stress. As stress builds, it creates anxiety, leading to self-doubts, particularly if a situation affects a man's public or job image. Erectile dysfunction can follow a career crisis. It can also be due to years of pressure to succeed and manage increasingly complex situations with more responsibilities. Career stress affecting sexual ability, though, is more often due to feelings of failure after layoffs, being passed over for a promotion, seeing younger people take over, lost opportunities, unfulfilling retirement, or demotions (especially those that imply a man is past his career prime). These blows hurt men in multiple ways because stress affects physical health and vitality, even lowering testosterone levels if prolonged. Depression sets in as a man anguishes over the hard work he put into getting to where he is and thinks about how he's eventually going to lose some or all of it.

A man loses his confidence because his self-image and male identity are tied closely to work. The results often play out in the bedroom. Stress and anxiety, combined with feelings of hopelessness, undermine his ability to relax or enjoy sex. As worries inhibit arousal, erection becomes harder to achieve. If an episode of erection failure threatens the already wounded ego, he's at risk for beginning a vicious circle of sexual dysfunction. When one sexual failure creates anxiety and embarrassment, the next time he tries he can fall into the trap of spectatoring (see the section "Spectatoring" later in this chapter).

Treatments for stress and depression include books such as *Feeling Good* by David Burns, support groups, self-examination of one's life, professional and spiritual counseling, or obtaining medication from a physician. Be aware, though, that many tranquilizers, antianxiety drugs, and antidepressants can themselves cause erectile difficulties. Ask your physician about side effects and other options.

Factors related to your wife.   Most women don't comprehend the influence they have over a man's spirit. It's amazing that some men function sexually at all in light of the difficult circumstances they deal with every day with their wives. Ironically, most of these women are loving, intelligent people with a blind spot on their otherwise tender hearts when it comes to honoring their husbands' sexual needs.

1. **She's not as attractive as she should be.** Some say the most important thing a man values about his wife is how physically attractive she is. Indeed, we know the first thing that draws two people to each other is their impression of each other's appearance. Once married, we must still work at remaining attractive to our spouses. Admittedly, age affects everyone, and we're not responsible for factors beyond our control, such as normal weight gain, graying hair, wrinkling skin, and so forth.

   Some women really let themselves go, though, putting little effort into maximizing what they still have. Such women show a lack of respect for themselves and their husbands. Many of these women suffer from depression. Unfortunately, it's difficult for a husband to tell his wife he would like her to look better without her becoming so defensive and hurt that she erupts in tears or anger. A more effective approach is to tell her how beautiful she is when she does put out some effort. Smart husbands continue to compliment their wives throughout life and show appreciation for their efforts. If your wife shows signs of depression, help her get professional treatment.

   If, on the other hand, your wife is already trying to be as attractive as possible, but you're unable to get past the fact that she is overweight/wrinkled/gray/whatever, you need to redefine feminine sexiness in terms that are ageless. A woman is sexy because her body is shaped differently than a man's, she has different anatomical parts, she acts loving and inviting, and she lets you know she thinks you're the greatest. You may find that the root of your erection problems is not in how your wife looks but rather in your own feelings of sexual unattractiveness and lost youth.

2. **She kills your spirit.** It's incredible how malicious some wives are toward their husbands.

   Bobbi constantly ridicules me for everything—from the way I dress, to how little money I make, how insignificant my accomplishments are, how clumsy or sloppy I am, what losers my friends and relatives are, to any insult you can imagine. Then she wonders why I can't feel loving and get turned on in bed after being treated like that all day.

Your wife may think she's making you into a better person, but she has no idea how destructive her words and attitudes are. Maybe she's a bitter woman who has fallen out of love. In either case, you both need marital counseling. Your lives will be miserable until you resolve the deep issues underlying her behavior, their effect on you, and your tolerance or mishandling of it. Until then there is little hope for a satisfying sexual relationship. Only as the marriage improves can the sexual side of it also mend.

3. **She's unresponsive.** Recently a woman in her late twenties told me she could get along without having sex for the rest of her life. The unfortunate men who find themselves married to such women discover before long that all the effort is one-sided as they struggle alone to keep their marital sex lives going. Their wives don't initiate sex, don't respond well to their husbands' advances, act as if they're doing their husbands a big favor when they do "give in," and may even belittle them for still wanting sex. These women have either lost their sex drive or have deep-seated sexual problems. Both partners need to read chapter 3 and would benefit from professional help to recapture her desire for sex.

   If you find yourself married to a woman like this, don't let her convince you that you're a perverted old man for having sexual feelings and needs—even if you're ninety years old. Sex between a husband and wife is an honorable act and an essential ingredient for a healthy marriage. Don't let her behavior be an excuse for you to look for sex with another woman, either. That would only create more problems by producing guilt, breaking trust, and risking the introduction of sexually transmitted diseases. Instead, face the problem together and get help.

4. **She's too holy for sex.** There was a time when the Roman Catholic Church held the belief that the only purpose of sex was procreation. Those days are history, and that church now believes that sex is also for pleasurable expression of love between a husband and wife. Nevertheless, there are women of every religion who believe or act like sex is a sinful, dirty act—even with their husbands. They are often unsympathetic and unresponsive to their husbands' sexual needs and may even condemn their husbands' natural, God-given sex drive. If a

woman convinces her husband that his normal urges are wrong, he'll experience shame whenever he feels them. He will develop difficulty achieving erections or becoming aroused enough to have intercourse. This is perfectly satisfactory to the wife, but it destroys his self-worth and the proper place of sex within marriage.

One of the best places to begin dealing with this problem is your nearest religious bookstore. There are several good books available now by religious authors who guide couples through the beauty of matrimonial sex. Often women of this type need counseling, too, perhaps by a clergyperson comfortable with the subject, or with a counselor who holds the same religious faith. Underlying her problem is often a background in which her parents stifled her with teachings centered on the evils and misuse of sex, while failing to glorify it as a natural and normal part of human love.

My mother had been sexually abused as a child and had seen a lot of it in our relatives' families, too. After she grew up, she became very religious, which did help her to forgive her father and gain strength from God. However, she thought the best way to teach me about sex was to tell me the horror stories of her life, I guess to make me careful around men so nothing bad would happen to me, too. I agreed that sex should be saved for marriage, but also absorbed the message that sex was evil. That carried over into my own marriage for many years.

Related to this problem is another one called "the Madonna-prostitute complex." In this, a man has erectile difficulty because *he* is the one who believes that sex is a dirty act. As a result he is able to perform sexually only with women he does not respect. He may see his wife as a proper maternal figure whom he cannot "defile," but he has no sexual difficulty with a prostitute or a "loose" woman. This man also needs professional counseling.

5. **She comes on too strongly.** As many women have become more liberated and have learned to ask for what they need rather than waiting for it to happen, some intimidate men by forcefully coming on to them. This problem is twofold. A man may want to take a leadership role in sex and, when he is

denied that, cannot then perform as a follower. Another man may have erectile difficulty with an aggressive woman because her style interferes with his ability to relax and enjoy the moment. These women usually operate out of ignorance. It simply won't work to demand that a man "perform." That type of pressure prevents the physiological process necessary for erection and orgasm. This is not to say that an occasional playful "attack" by a wife who obviously enjoys her husband's sexuality is wrong. Most men relish the occasional turnabout of roles if their wives do so with a frisky approach that doesn't demand that he "put out" for her.

Boredom.　On the average, men prefer more and different sexual techniques than do women. While boredom is more likely to create marital dissatisfaction than sexual dysfunction, boredom can build into resentment that inhibits sexual arousal. Also, it's perfectly normal for men (and women, too) to need "a little something extra" to boost sexual arousal after years and years of doing the same thing in the same way with the same person.

It's much better to pursue variety with your wife than to pursue a variety of sexual partners. If you want to expand your sexual repertoire, show your wife the following list. Each of you should use a separate answer sheet to avoid affecting each other's responses. Share them only when finished. The discussion that follows this exercise often opens doors of exploration that you as a couple may not try otherwise. Perhaps you each assumed the other person wouldn't like a certain activity, so you never mentioned it. Activities listed below are safe and appropriate between married partners. There are many more techniques beyond these, intentionally omitted if they are health or safety risks.

Fun and Games for Married Couples

Next to each activity listed below that you and your spouse have *never done* together, write "Yes," "No," or "Maybe" to indicate your willingness to try it. For each activity you and your spouse have *already tried* with each other, give it a grade.

A:　You really enjoyed it.
B:　It was pleasant, but you want to do it only occasionally.
C:　You could take it or leave it.

D: It was unappealing, but you would do it again if your spouse liked it.

E: It was such a turnoff that you don't want to do it again for at least five years.

When finished (and not until then!), share your answers with your spouse.

1. _____ Nipple stimulation of your spouse
2. _____ Nipple stimulation by your spouse
3. _____ Manual stimulation of the clitoris
4. _____ Manual stimulation of the penis
5. _____ French kissing
6. _____ Sex outdoors
7. _____ Woman-on-top intercourse position
8. _____ Intercourse from behind (penis in the vagina, not anal entry)
9. _____ Sex in the kitchen, living room, shower, etc. (specify a place: _____)
10. _____ A planned weekend away just for romance and sex
11. _____ A spontaneous weekend away just for romance and sex
12. _____ Watching an erotic videotape
13. _____ Doing a striptease or erotic dance for your spouse
14. _____ Watching your spouse do a striptease or erotic dance
15. _____ Sex standing up
16. _____ Sex in the car
17. _____ Using a vibrator
18. _____ Using a dildo or other sex toy
19. _____ Reading sexy literature with or aloud to your spouse
20. _____ Putting his finger into her vagina
21. _____ Having your earlobes kissed
22. _____ Getting a total body massage
23. _____ Sucking your spouse's toes
24. _____ Giving each other oral sex simultaneously ("69")

25. _____ Candlelight during sex
26. _____ Your spouse wearing sexy lingerie or under
wear
27. _____ Wearing sexy lingerie or underwear
28. _____ Discovering your spouse is wearing no under
wear
29. _____ Using incense, perfume, scented oils, etc. (your
ideas: _____)
30. _____ Watching your spouse masturbate
31. _____ Masturbating in front of your spouse
32. _____ Taking a shower or bath together
33. _____ Making out in the back row at a movie
34. _____ Attending a marriage enrichment seminar
35. _____ Dressing up like a fantasy character for sex
(specify: _____)
36. _____ Fellatio (oral sex performed on the husband)
37. _____ Cunnilingus (oral sex performed on the wife)
38. _____ "Intercourse" between the breasts
39. _____ Just the two of you dancing at home alone
40. _____ Just the two of you dancing at home alone
naked
41. _____ Taking nude photos of each other
42. _____ Being kidnapped by your spouse for an erotic
outing
43. _____ Sex during a menstrual period
44. _____ Stroking of the scrotum
45. _____ Licking whipped cream (other food, specify:
_____) off each other
46. _____ Having sex in an elevator
47. _____ Reading a sex manual together
48. _____ Giving little nibbling bites
49. _____ Getting little nibbling bites
50. _____ Having ice stroked on your penis/tummy/clit-
oris/nipples, etc. (specify: _____)
51. _____ Watching yourselves have sex in a mirror
52. _____ Sitting in a hot tub together
53. _____ Having sex in a hot tub
54. _____ Shampooing your spouse's hair
55. _____ Getting a shampoo from your spouse
56. _____ Experimenting with nontraditional intercourse
positions (ideas: _____)

57. _____ Hearing more moaning, screaming, or sexy talk

58. _____ Doing more moaning, screaming, or sexy talk

59. _____ Hot and hard and deep intercourse

60. _____ Soft and tender intercourse

61. _____ Telling each other your sexual fantasies

62. _____ Putting a finger in your spouse's anus during sex

63. _____ Getting a finger put in your anus during sex

64. _____ Anal intercourse

Add your own ideas here: _____

_____

Spectatoring. Chapter 3 covered the basic issues surrounding the problem of spectatoring. There are, however, other aspects that pertain especially to men. Men are more likely to fall into the trap of spectatoring because, while women can fake orgasms, men cannot fake erections, and they feel great pressure to produce them. The body is generally incapable of becoming sexually aroused, particularly to the point of orgasm, though, when the mind is anxious and the body is tense.

Since the reason for erectile failure sometimes remains a mystery, there is often little a man can consciously do to prevent it from happening again. He can improve his chances of better sexual performance by avoiding alcohol, tobacco, overeating, and fatigue, but other than that, he usually can do little more. As if from a distance, he then watches himself to see how well he does. This inhibits relaxation, making it easier to fail again. As a result he's likely to feel shame and embarrassment, compounding the problem even more. The more anxious he is going into his next sexual encounter, the more likely he is to fail again. He may keep score as if he were a spectator at a sports event, monitoring how often he has sex and how often he is successful.

Women aren't oblivious to their husbands' erectile difficulties. A careful wife does the best she can to preserve her husband's self-esteem, assuring him he is just having a hard time tonight or is under a lot of stress right now. She shouldn't make a big deal out of it, should probably not talk about it at great length, and should bolster her husband's ego in other ways. The wife who observes that her husband's sexual dysfunction is increasing, though, may feel frustration as she watches as a helpless bystander, wishing she could do something but not knowing what. Some women in this situation pretend to lose interest in sex to avoid embarrassing their husbands further by not putting them in the position of having to face the problem. This is not a solution. In fact, this can be the death sentence of the couple's sex life if they don't start communicating.

> *A couple of years ago Nettie and I could have been characters in an O. Henry story. Things were really getting to me at work: my new boss had cut the number of managers in half, which essentially doubled my workload, not to mention that he was a real schmuck. The upshot was that I was so stressed and angry all the time, it started to affect my energy. Okay, I'll admit it: I was depressed. I had thought that job was going to be my ticket to retirement, but I didn't know how I was going to hold on seven more years like that. I started having trouble performing in bed. I knew what was wrong, but I wanted to hide it from Nettie so she wouldn't worry. Little did I know, she was already worried but wanted to hide her concern from me. She thought if she mentioned my sexual problem, it would embarrass me too much and make things worse. So she started acting like she wasn't interested in sex anymore, just to save my feelings. There we were, neither of us acting like we wanted sex, but both of us too worried to admit to the game we were playing. What finally broke the ice was when I came home from work one day and just blew up. I couldn't take it anymore. We took the phone off the hook and spent that whole night talking out everything—our goals, our problems, our marriage. After that things seemed better, even though it took a few weeks to make the changes needed.*

To halt the spectatoring, the first thing a couple must do is stop having sex for a while. This takes pressure off the husband to perform and allows the sex drive to build. Then the couple should proceed through the sensate focusing and nondemand pleasuring exercises discussed in chapter 3. While the context there is for a woman with sexual difficulty, the techniques work the same for men. When you get to genital massage, the man should lie flat on his back with his legs separated and have his wife sit between them, facing him with her knees over his thighs. He should direct her to do what feels good to him. Clearly understand that the purpose of this exercise is not to bring him to orgasm or to have intercourse. If he has an erection, he can enjoy it but otherwise ignore it. If there is no erection at this point, that's fine, too. He should just relax, pay attention to the sensations, and know he is under no obligation to do anything except feel pleasure.

If you find these exercises are enjoyable and increase your intimacy, but don't eventually lead to reestablishment of erectile and orgasmic function, it's time to seek professional help. Start first with a complete physical and sexual examination by a qualified physician to rule out anything physically wrong. Then find a certified sex therapist. It is often difficult to admit you need professional help. Know, though, that the chances for success are excellent. The professionals who will work with you are discreet. You needn't continue suffering with this problem. Even if standard treatments and therapies don't work, there's still hope through medications, mechanical devices, or surgery to reestablish your erectile ability. Avoid taking those steps, though, until you have thoroughly investigated the physical and psychological causes and given less extreme measures an opportunity to work.

Physical Causes of Erectile Dysfunction

Just as the list of reasons for why erection problems may be psychological is lengthy, the list of physical causes is long, too, and growing rapidly. Here we will look at a few of the possible causes, leaving others for upcoming chapters.

Respiratory problems that cause fatigue. There are many illnesses that occur more frequently in men that contribute to fatigue, such as smoking-related problems. Men who smoke outnumber the women who do. It's likely that a man with a long history of smoking will have breathing difficulty and shortness of breath. Any condition that makes oxygen exchange in the lungs harder or inhibits full lung expansion, such as emphysema, requires sexual adjustment. The man with emphysema may have more energy in the morning than at night, but he is also more likely to need an hour or two upon rising to empty his lungs of secretions so he can breathe more easily. Therefore he might tolerate sex better in the early afternoon.

Regardless of what respiratory problem exacerbates fatigue, new intercourse positions become necessary to allow maximum lung expansion and prevent shortness of breath that often comes while lying flat in bed. Better positions for intercourse include any that allow him to sit upright, perhaps using pillows or innovative seated positions. The key here is to feel total freedom to do whatever is necessary to make sex comfortable for you and your partner.

> One technique we discovered, only because we were getting really frustrated over my emphysema preventing us from enjoying sex in bed, involved an old rocking chair we keep on the back porch. One afternoon I was sitting out there reading when I felt Donna's arms around me from behind. She then came around front, unzipped my pants, pulled out my penis, and played with me a little until I was hard. I never had to move. Then she pulled up her dress (she had no underwear on!) and sat down facing me, working me inside her as she lowered herself onto my lap. That old chair doesn't have any arms on it, so it worked pretty well. She held on to the back of it, and I hung on to the barbecue on one side and the doghouse on the other side. We just rocked away into ecstasy. It was great because it didn't leave me wrung out. I could still sit up and get my breath the whole time.

Back pain from muscle strain.   Most pain occurs after a man injures muscles in his lower back. The strain comes from abdominal weight gain, poor posture, improper lifting techniques, or twisting motions. The best treatment is to take pain relievers to reduce the pain, apply a heating pad, avoid further strain, and stay on bed rest for a day or so while lying in a position that curves the lower back outward (as when the knees are brought toward the chest). However, the position a man finds most comfortable for his back may make intercourse impossible. Many intercourse positions couples traditionally use put greater stress on the man's back than the woman's.

Prior to having sex during a flare-up of back trouble, the husband would be wise to take an analgesic at least thirty to sixty minutes in advance and warn his wife that he may need to change his position if a muscle spasm starts. Typically, back problems from muscle strain last only a few days, so if a couple decides intercourse is not worth the effort, they can just abstain temporarily until the pain subsides. They can creatively enjoy orgasm through manual stimulation or oral sex, saving intercourse for another day. When his back feels better, a man must continue to guard against using sexual techniques that risk reinjury. Therefore he should avoid intercourse positions that require standing, that support his wife's weight with his arms, or that make him stick his stomach out (this may put back muscles into spasm).

Substance abuse. Alcohol is deadly to sexual function. It suppresses nerve impulses and diminishes the quality of nerve messages sent through the sexual reflex arc via the spinal cord to the pelvic organs. Alcohol decreases the firmness of erections and prolongs the excitement phase of male sexual response.

If a man continues to increase his alcohol consumption as the years pass and finds that he needs more drinks to accomplish the same level of relaxation or mental anesthesia, he needs to evaluate his priorities. Chronic overuse of alcohol not only destroys sexual function, it also is associated with shrinkage of the testes and decreased production of testosterone. The sex drive declines and may even disappear. With less circulating testosterone, he starts to lose some of his male physical characteristics, looking more feminine as his breasts enlarge and his pubic hair becomes more sparse. Excessive alcohol also destroys other body organs, such as the liver and the brain, leading to general poor health and loss of sexual appeal to women. The solution is plain: get help to stop drinking.

Other substances cause erectile dysfunction, too. Any chemical that alters the mood toward euphoria or the depths of sedation affects a man's desire for sex and his ability to obtain an erection. Depressant drugs, both illicit and legal ones (such as Valium), deaden the libido as well as mental acuity. People who claim marijuana enhances sexual enjoyment are experiencing a placebo effect or a time perception distortion. Stimulants such as cocaine also destroy the libido within just a few trials. The rapidly addictive nature of these drugs creates such a craving for them that the normal desires of life, such as sex, become less important.

Few people realize how tobacco affects male sexual function beyond fatigue from respiratory problems. Nicotine absorbed during tobacco use has an immediate effect, and constricts blood vessels, including those to the penis. As less blood can flow into the penis, erection is more difficult, particularly if a man has used tobacco within thirty minutes before sex. The long-term result of nicotine is that arteriosclerosis, including the buildup of plaque along their inner walls (see below), prevents them from expanding efficiently enough to permit full penile engorgement. It also restricts blood flow as artery passageways narrow over the years. While it is very difficult to break the tobacco habit, a man who notices erectile difficulty should at least avoid using tobacco immediately prior to attempting sex.

Blood vessel and heart disease.   One of the most important causes of erectile dysfunction is arteriosclerosis or "hardening of the arteries," a problem that usually occurs earlier in men than women. In this, arteries accumulate a buildup of plaque and cholesterol, narrowing their inner diameter and limiting their flexibility. They are also not able to expand as well. As a result, blood cannot get through as easily. The heart works harder to pump blood through the narrowed vessels, using more pressure to push it into distant parts of the body needing oxygen. Medications for high blood pressure may interfere with erectile ability by preventing the retention of blood in the penis during sexual arousal.

Arteriosclerosis also affects erectile function by blocking the influx of blood into the penis. During sexual excitement not enough blood flows into the penis fast enough to exceed the rate of blood flowing out of it. Unfortunately, men hear very little about the risks of blood vessel disease in relation to sex.

> *Man, it blew me away when I heard my high cholesterol was causing my penis problems! I'd known for years I was overweight and needed to stop smoking, but I figured when it's time for me to go, I'll go. All I ever heard was, "You're on the road to a heart attack or a stroke." If somebody had told me it would also plug up the arteries to my penis, I'd have done something about it a lot sooner!*

For complete information on blood vessel and heart disease related to sexual function, see chapter 9.

Diabetes.   Diabetes is another physical cause of erectile dysfunction that we see more frequently than before. Insulin-dependent diabetes ("Type I diabetes") is a disease in which a person doesn't produce enough insulin, a substance necessary for the body's cells to use sugar. It often appears before age thirty. Type II diabetes usually occurs after age fifty as older people gain weight, their bodies use sugar less efficiently, and they make less insulin. There's no cure yet for either type of diabetes, but current treatments

successfully prolong most diabetics' lives well past their reproductive years. Hence more diabetics are living long enough to experience the long-term effects of this disease on sexual function.
Since diabetes can be hereditary and since more people with diabetes are living long enough to have children, this also adds to
the greater number of people in the population with diabetes.

The impact of diabetes on erectile ability is significant, so
much so that when any man has erectile difficulty and comes to
his physician, a test for diabetes is always wise. Many new cases
of diabetes are first discovered from the presenting symptom of
erectile failure. The longer a man has had diabetes, the more
likely it is he'll develop difficulty with erections. A majority of diabetic men over sixty years of age have erectile dysfunction. Men
who developed diabetes at a younger age have more sexual difficulty as they get older than do men the same age they are but
who've had diabetes for a shorter time.

Diabetes-related erectile dysfunction is probably due to
two factors. First, the disease gradually damages nerves throughout the body, including those supplying pelvic and genital
organs. Sexual implications include loss of penile sensation,
nerve response promoting erection, and orgasmic ability.

One test for erectile dysfunction related to diabetic nerve damage is to evaluate whether there has been a concurrent loss of
bladder sensation. If a diabetic man has trouble recognizing when
his bladder is full or has poor urine control, this may be a clue
that his erectile problems are also due to diabetes-related nerve
damage. Since nerves cannot be repaired, there's no way to cure
loss of sensation to the bladder or penis. Women with diabetes
may experience progressive numbness of their genitals, too, so
that they need more intense clitoral stimulation to reach orgasm.

A diabetic man may notice that nerves that promote an erection no longer function well but that nerves that receive and send
tactile massages do. In this case he may still be capable of having
orgasms without erections. If he wants to have intercourse, he's
going to have to use assistive devices or erection-producing medications.

Another variation is that a diabetic man may have an orgasm
with or without erection, but not ejaculate. This is because nerves
controlling the internal sphincter muscles at the bottom of his
bladder are malfunctioning. His ejaculation is forced back up into
his bladder rather than out through the penis. The next time he

urinates after orgasm, his urine looks cloudy because it contains semen. Retrograde ejaculation is not harmful but renders him incapable of impregnating a woman without medical assistance.

The second possible reason for why diabetes affects erection is that most diabetics develop circulatory problems, shown by how much harder it is for wounds to heal. Impaired circulation and plugging of penile arteries cause the same problems mentioned with arteriosclerosis. The solutions are also generally the same, since many diabetics also have artery disease and high blood pressure.

> *About five years ago my diabetes really started taking a toll on my body. I'd been having more trouble getting erections. It finally reached a point where I never had them at all. It was pretty obvious to Estelle, of course. One day I just broke down and cried like a baby and told her I'd failed her as a husband. When she heard what was bothering me, she said (I'll never forget this), "Oh, is that all? Well, frankly, it's a big relief to me. I never liked sex anyway." She might as well have shot me through the head. It killed something important in me. I was hoping we could look for solutions together, because while my plumbing wasn't working, my head still was—meaning I still felt a strong sex drive. After that, though, I just gave up.*

Because there's no cure for diabetes, the best way to slow loss of sexual function is to control the progression of the disease. Control of blood sugar levels by complying with dietary, exercise, and medication regimens is the only way to accomplish that. If erectile problems or loss of penile sensations begin to appear, it's time to consider other mechanisms for achieving orgasm or intercourse. In the case of a man whose penis has become relatively numb, he won't regain all of the physical pleasure of penile stimulation he once enjoyed. However, he can resume intercourse by turning to penile implants and erection-promoting devices and medications.

Other types of nerve degeneration or damage.   Nerve disorders originate in four possible locations: in the brain, in the spinal cord, as a generalized progressive neuromuscular disease, or in specific local nerves during surgery or accidents. Disorders in the brain that become more likely with age are Parkinson's disease, Alzheimer's disease, and cerebrovascular accidents (strokes). All of these can cause softer or shorter-lasting erections or erratic loss of erectile ability. They also affect other aspects of sexuality; therefore we'll address these problems in chapter 10.

Spinal cord function is extremely important to male sexuality because nerve reflex arcs to and from the spinal cord control erection. Men who have suffered a spinal cord injury, who have had spinal cord compression, whose back surgery involved cutting of nerves, or even men with a herniated vertebral disk can have sexual problems that require individualized evaluation. For example, unless spinal cord function is completely disrupted at some point along its length, some nerves may continue to work well while others do not. This means that one man who has lost partial use of his lower body may still be capable of having an erection, while another man's erections may be unpredictable or may occur independent of penile stimulation. Orgasm may be spontaneous as well. The brain might be able to sense penile stimulation but the reflex arc through the spinal cord may not function properly, preventing erection or orgasm. Since these problems also affect more than just erectile ability, refer to chapter 10 for more information.

Several diseases with a generalized effect gradually cause erection problems. For example, approximately 50 percent of men with multiple sclerosis have erectile dysfunction. Men with neuromuscular disorders are candidates for penile devices and erection medications, but also need to adapt intercourse positions and sexual techniques as they lose muscle function in other body parts. They may also find that muscle relaxants or other therapies are helpful for preventing muscle spasms that seem worse during sexual arousal. Many men with these problems discover that certain times of day or even certain days are better than others for sexual success.

Any time a man has surgery in the lower abdomen or pelvis, there is risk of cutting or traumatizing nerves supplying the genitals. Surgeries notorious for doing this are colectomy, colostomy, and removal of the prostate in a manner that requires a surgical incision instead of getting to it via the urinary tube. For information on these procedures see chapters 7 and 8.

Kidney disease. Short-term urine or kidney infections don't affect sexual ability. However, with chronic kidney (renal) disease, erectile dysfunction may become progressively worse as kidneys fail. Not every man with kidney disease has erection problems. Chronic kidney disease does produce progressive weakness, fatigue, and slower mental processes because the body retains toxins, fluid, and sodium. Kidneys don't clear medications as well as they should, and allow protein to escape the body. Because water and sodium increase, blood pressure rises and the heart works harder. As the disease continues, blood vessel changes can affect erectile ability. Kidney disease is often related to hyperprolactinemia, an elevation of the hormone prolactin made in the brain that causes erectile and thyroid dysfunction.

The psychological impact of renal disease is doubly difficult, not only because erectile function may decline, but also because a man may eventually have to rely on kidney dialysis. This is a procedure performed every two to three days in which a special machine filters all of the body's blood, clearing it of toxins and excess fluids. It's a life-saving measure; without it he would die. However, it does mean that his penis may not only lose some sexual function, it also ceases to be necessary for urination. The psychological impact of depending on a dialysis machine can also be emasculating.

> *The dialysis center nearest to where we live is 125 miles away. It takes us two hours to get there if the traffic isn't bad. It takes about an hour to get checked in and set up, then I'm attached to the machine for three hours. Another hour goes by waiting for the staff to wrap up everything and getting back on the road. That's nine hours out of my life every Tuesday, Thursday, and Saturday for dialysis. Every night before I'm due to go back, I'm wasted because the toxins are building up in my blood, and I'm really tired and can't think straight. What kind of a life is this? Well, it's a life full of financial worries because I can't really hold down a job. It's a strain on my wife because she has to go with me to dialysis and takes care of me the rest of the time. It takes a lot of humility for me to know I'm so sick and have to depend on her so much for things a mother would normally do, not a wife. We just live in constant hope for a phone call from the organ donor bank saying they have a kidney for me.*

Since kidney dialysis takes several hours and disrupts life so completely, it's no wonder most people seek organ transplants. The sexual outlook is very hopeful for those who obtain a new kidney. Most men by far regain lost sexual ability within a couple of years after a kidney transplant.

Without a transplant, loss of sexual desire caused by hormonal imbalances and psychological factors is difficult to combat. Physical energy required to cope with kidney disease and frequent dialysis also robs a couple of sexual energy. They must talk frankly and maximize remaining function. For example, many people feel almost normal the morning after dialysis, an ideal time to take advantage of better strength for sex.

Hormonal imbalances. Anything that upsets one part of the hormone system can upset other parts. For example, whenever a man's thyroid gland produces less than the normal amount of hormone, he eventually produces less testosterone, too. Follicle-stimulating hormone (FSH) and luteinizing hormone (LH) are female hormones that the male brain also produces in small amounts. Abnormally high levels of these substances also affect sexual desire and function. Low testosterone, of course, is the most significant hormone affecting the sex drive and can result from a wide variety of possible causes.

The good news about hormonal imbalances is that usually they are reversible. If the body is low on a particular hormone, a man can use a prescription to replace it. If the level is too high, the treatment is more complicated, because the physician must remove or suppress the tissue that is making too much of it. The most challenging hormone to replace is testosterone, since the easiest way to take it (as a pill) renders most of it worthless because digestion destroys it. Furthermore, some physicians believe it promotes liver damage.

Better options include getting an injection of testosterone every two to three weeks, wearing a skin patch containing testosterone cream, or using special tablets that dissolve under the tongue for direct absorption into the bloodstream. By the way, testosterone does not boost the sex drive if it already exists in normal amounts. It is not an aphrodisiac. Furthermore, taking testosterone in any form is risky because it can accelerate the risk of heart attacks and strokes and the growth of preexisting prostate cancer.

Medications. Many legal drugs can affect libido, erectile function, or ejaculation. If you discover you're taking a medication on the following list, don't discontinue it without discussing options with your physician. After all, worse things can happen if you stop taking an important medicine than losing some sexual ability—such as having a heart attack! Here's a partial list of medications that have affected male sexuality (some of these categories and drugs overlap, but are listed in this manner to help you recognize certain ones more easily):

adrenergics

amitriptyline (Elavil)

anticholinergics

antidepressants

antihypertensives

atropine

benzodiazepines

beta blockers

calcium channel blockers

cancer chemotherapeutics

chlorpromazine (Thorazine)

cimetidine (Tagamet)

clofibrate (Atromid)

decongestants

digitalis (Digoxin)

disulfiram (Antabuse)

fluoxetine (Prozac)

haloperidol (Haldol)

imipramine (Tofranil)

lithium

many drugs used to treat
    prostate cancer

metronidazole (Flagyl)

phenothiazines

prescription narcotics (mor-
    phine, codeine, Demerol)

sedatives, hypnotics

some seizure medications

sympatholytics

synthetic progesterones
    (Depo-Provera)

thioridazine (Mellaril)

tranquilizers

A word of caution is appropriate here. Anything, including a medication, that you *think* will hurt your sexual performance will! (Also, anything you believe will help you sexually has a good chance of improving your sex life, too—even if it's a worthless sugar pill.) This is the "placebo" effect, which means your expectations are a powerful determinant of a drug's effect. Therefore, avoid prejudging whether a medicine will alter your sexual potential. Many of these listed alter function in only a minority of men. Give your medicine a fair trial and try to be objective about the results.

Terminal illness.   The loss of energy and normal function that occurs as death approaches almost always depletes a man's sexual desire and ability. Most men who are terminally ill also experience a psychological blow to their self-esteem when faced with loss of control and self-determination that define them as male beings. A couple confronting death of the husband can choose to go down this road supporting each other or to become more isolated and withdrawn. A wife must find ways to keep her husband feeling as masculine as possible, helping him to make important contributions in whatever ways he finds meaningful, both within the sexual relationship and in daily life. If his male identity is not preserved, psychological effects will predate effects of physical illness on sexual function.

A couple should hang on to sexuality as long as possible and adapt their strategies as often as necessary for that to happen. Near the end only the wife may be orgasming, but her husband can hold her while she masturbates and share in her pleasure by sending sexual messages and love. She can release him from guilt for not doing more. He can give her permission to pursue her sexual fulfillment after he dies. When the end is near, erectile function is no longer very important. What matters much more is that sexuality can be defined in terms of love and companionship and intimacy.

Penile Devices, Drugs, Procedures, and Implants

Many "remedies" claim to improve a man's "potency," such as Spanish fly, cantharidine, rhinoceros horn powder, ginseng, and so forth. They assert that hard and longer-lasting erections are only a phone call away. The truth is, though, that many devices and potions fail to live up to their advertising, and some can actually hurt you. Their side effects can be toxic, or they can severely damage your penis. There's certainly nothing a man who has satisfactory sexual function can gain from such methods.

However, if your erectile disability has become severe and your physician hasn't pinpointed a cause (or if the cause is irreversible), you may want to consider the following options. *Be aware that although all of these promote or even guarantee erections, they won't restore orgasms or ejaculation if you've lost those abilities due to diabetes or nerve damage.* However, if your loss of orgasm is psychologically related to the fact that you're physically unable to have an erection, being able to have erections again may be so rewarding to you that your ability to orgasm also returns.

Many men use the following methods even if they can never restore orgasmic ability, though, because having intercourse is so important to their self-esteem. Intercourse is also important because it preserves a vital part of many couples' sexual relationship. Some wives are pleased their husbands opt for therapies to restore erectile ability because they, too, miss that aspect of sex.

> *I would never have admitted this to Ira ahead of time, but I was thrilled when he decided to get his penile implant. He's a great husband and continued to attend to my sexual needs after his surgery for prostate cancer when he lost his erections. I missed intercourse, though. There's such an emotional bond between us during it that having sex only on "the outside parts" lacks. He's like a young man again now. He's so cute and tickled with himself every time he pumps up his implant. Sometimes he pumps it up just for fun, hooting just like those guys on Saturday Night Live who say, "We are going to PUMP YOU UP!"*

Restoring erectile function through mechanical or medicinal means is an extremely important topic for a couple to discuss thoroughly before taking radical or expensive measures. They must be absolutely honest with each other about whether erection and intercourse are essential to their sexual happiness. Let's examine the factors they should consider.

Pills

1. **Yohimbine.** Yohimbine (Yocun) has a long history of unsubstantiated aphrodisiacal claims, but it may have some ability to enhance erection. It is a nonprescription derivative of the bark of a West African tree. Yohimbine acts primarily as a placebo, although it does produce dilation of some blood vessels. This results in a flushed feeling, but some men say it also opens their penile vessels, causing erection. Yohimbine blocks norepinephrine release, a natural body chemical that constricts blood vessels. When norepinephrine doesn't act, smooth muscles in artery walls relax and open wider, increasing blood flow. Yohimbine isn't effective in most cases, though. At best, erections are rather soft in quality.

2. **Trazodone.** Some men who take trazodone for depression report it improves erectile ability. Treating depression itself often results in improved sexual interest, but trazodone also acts chemically to inhibit the body's use of serotonin, a strong blood vessel constrictor. This increases blood flow into the

spongy bodies of the penis (the corpora cavernosa and the corpus spongiosum). A few men have developed erections that lasted well beyond orgasm and could not get their erections to subside. This condition, called priapism, constitutes an emergency (see chapter 5).

3. **Apomorphine.** Apomorphine is a prescription pill dissolved under the tongue for direct absorption into circulation. It affects the brain region associated with erections by chemically acting on dopamine, a forerunner of norepinephrine, the blood vessel constrictor mentioned earlier. Originally veterinarians used apomorphine to induce vomiting in animals, but its effect on erection made it of interest in human medicine as well. The erections it produces are of fairly good quality. However, nausea can be a serious side effect.

4. **Viagra.** Even though it is quite expensive, sildenafil citrate (Viagra) is attractive because men don't have to take it continuously and it has few side effects. It doesn't bring about erections unless the penis is stimulated, making it more desirable than drugs such as apomorphine or trazodone. One pill taken about an hour before intercourse quite effectively blocks an enzyme (phosphodiesterase) that decreases penile blood flow. It works best if not taken with high-fat foods.

   Some men have erections the next morning, too, without taking an additional pill. This is because, while the medicine clears from the blood in a few hours, penile tissues may harbor some of it a little longer. Such erections are useful for intercourse, too.

   Not every man finds Viagra to be the answer, but it is successful in about 66 percent of cases of erectile dysfunction. It does nothing to improve the quality of sexual performance of a man who already has satisfactory erectile ability.

   Possible side effects include headache, flushing, or stomach upset. You can take a pain reliever or antacid for these problems. Many men report these problems become less severe over time. Another side effect involves changes in color vision. Viagra can make men see a blue haze or perceive light as being more bright than usual while the medicine is in their systems. This is because the enzyme it blocks in the penis is similar to an enzyme in the retina. This side effect is not dangerous and does not harm the eyes.

Men who are on nitrate heart medicines such as nitroglycerin, Imdur, Isordil, or nitroprusside should not take Viagra
because it enhances the arterial dilation effect, causing greater
risk of dropping blood pressure, fainting, and even death. Any
man who starts Viagra needs to stay within his physical fitness limits as he tries out his renewed sexual potential, to
avoid overexerting to the point of heart strain, particularly
men recovering from a heart attack or a stroke. Sudden death
from overexertion while on Viagra occurs rarely but can be
avoided. If vessel dilation anywhere in the body would present a problem for any reason, Viagra is not recommended.

Injections.   To work properly, some medications must be injected directly into the penis. These are prescription drugs, and
include papaverine (with or without phentolamine) or Caverject
(a prostaglandin). They, too, primarily promote blood flow into
the penis by relaxing artery wall muscles.

A man interested in trying an injectable erectile stimulant
starts by practicing giving himself the medicine as his physician
watches and teaches him. The man inserts a thin needle almost
half an inch into one of the corpora cavernosa, the spongy bodies that run the length of the penis, and presses the plunger on
the syringe to inject the medicine. The erection appears quickly
and can last up to ninety minutes, although most last about thirty
minutes. The erection produced is fairly firm and quite rigid. Often the physician must adjust the dosage, requiring more than
one appointment.

Disadvantages include overcoming squeamishness about inserting the needle, possible penile pain, the risk of uncontrollably
long erections, and the possibility of scarring with long-term use.
Scarring inside the corpora cavernosa can render a penis incapable of full expansion, or may cause a twisted appearance of the
penis because scar tissue doesn't stretch well during engorgement. Few men realize that with this method erections don't subside after orgasm. The medication must wear off.

Suppositories.   Another option is alprostadil (Muse), a prostaglandin that relaxes artery walls, letting blood flow into the penis
faster than it flows out. Muse comes with a disposable insertion
instrument that allows a man to put a tiny pellet of medication

into the urinary opening at the tip of his penis. The pellet is about one-quarter-inch long and about one-sixteenth-inch thick. He learns how to push it one inch into the urinary tube, practicing at first in the physician's office. He should then sit or walk for about ten minutes, rather than lying down and trying to have sex immediately, to take advantage of gravity to pull blood into the penis while the medication starts to work. Erections last thirty to sixty minutes.

About a third of men who use Muse report pain in their genitals (particularly the penis), and many also have pain into the legs. About one out of ten men has a burning sensation in the urinary tube. Other, less common side effects include swelling of leg veins, dizziness, and fainting (because the drug can also relax arteries in the brain). Muse requires a prescription and sometimes two or three office visits to adjust the dosage.

The biggest complaint men have about this method is that the penile enlargement doesn't necessarily include rigidity, too. While the penis gets larger, it may not get as stiff and as hard as they like.

Vacuum devices.   Several men's magazines and pharmacies sell these devices, which consist of a plastic cylinder, closed at one end, attached to a pumping mechanism. The cylinder fits over the penis. The pump then removes the air, creating a vacuum that pulls blood into the penis from the body. Partial erection usually occurs in about five minutes. After removing the cylinder, the man must slip a constriction ring onto the penis, and roll it down to the base next to his body to keep blood in the penis as long as possible. It's extremely important to remove the constriction ring right after intercourse. Never leave it on more than a total of thirty minutes.

The erection produced is softer than normal and does not last long. While this is a rather cumbersome method, it doesn't require a prescription. If you try a vacuum device, you might notice the same effect a "hickey" produces because of the effect of suction on the skin. About half of all men develop petechiae (small red dots just under the skin where capillaries have broken). About a third have some bruising of their penis. Both symptoms gradually disappear in a few days unless you use the vacuum cylinder again.

Constriction rings ("tourniquets").   Constriction rings are not only useful with vacuum devices, but also alone. A constriction ring is a soft plastic circle similar to a stiff rubber band. Some rings have little wing-type handles, making removal easier in case the ring becomes lodged under a skin fold.

To apply the ring, the man slips it down over his penis to the very base. The ring works like a tourniquet by applying pressure, allowing blood to flow in through penile arteries that lie deeper inside the penis, but obstructing blood flow out through the veins that lie closer to the surface. The erection produced is semihard, but firm enough for intercourse.

Men have three primary complaints regarding this device. First, it can hurt. Putting it on requires a delicate touch, and a man must remove it while the penis is still erect, because the penis cannot disengorge while the ring is in place. Another complaint is that the ring renders the penis numb after a few minutes. This is because the ring compresses nerves as well as arteries, making the penis "fall asleep," just as your foot falls asleep when you've crossed your legs too long. Of course, when the penis is numb it cannot perceive stimulation as well. Therefore, this method makes intercourse possible, but isn't entirely satisfactory for achieving orgasms.

Third, engorgement takes place only from the band to the tip of the penis. It doesn't provide any erection behind the band at the base of the penis. Therefore the penis bends like a hinge at the base where it's softer, making some intercourse positions difficult.

Different sizes are available. Be careful not to let the one you use be too tight because that could cause cell damage. Remove the constriction ring as soon as possible. If you leave the ring on and fall asleep overnight, you could seriously damage your penis. (After all, this is one method farmers use to remove lambs' tails!)

I figured why spend twenty-five bucks on some gadget I could make out of a big rubber band? The first time I used a rubber band on my penis, though, I couldn't get it off. I was starting to hurt and got in too big of a hurry. The stupid thing was all wet and slippery and got tangled in my pubic hair. The longer it was on, the deeper it sank into the skin around my fat gut. I just couldn't get a grip on it. I was having trouble seeing over my stomach anyway and was starting to panic. Cheryl wasn't home at the time to help me (you figure it out). I didn't know what else to do so I drove to the emer-

gency room as fast as I could without attracting a cop (can you imagine trying to explain THAT?!). The doctor was able to get it off in no time. I ended up paying more for the emergency room visit than four of the gizmos out of the magazine would have cost me. After that, I tied a string to the rubber band first so I could find it easier later and pull it out enough to snip it with the scissors.

Penile implants. Many men like the idea of a penile implant because it sounds like an easy, long-term solution to erectile failure. However, implants require surgery, involve placing foreign materials into the body, and are quite expensive in relation to other solutions. The cost for the procedure, anesthesia, nursing care, office visits, the equipment, and so forth amounts to a few thousand dollars. Some men who still have the ability to orgasm, but lost it from being discouraged about their erectile dysfunction, may find that the cost is worth it because a penile implant renews their self-confidence and thus restores orgasms, too.

The man who undergoes this procedure will first need laboratory tests, a physical examination, and X rays several days in advance. He mustn't eat or drink for at least eight hours before the operation. He usually gets a general anesthetic, allowing him to sleep for the hour or so the operation takes. Recovery to full alertness takes several more hours. Therefore, he shouldn't expect to go home until late afternoon or the evening of the surgery. Some surgeons keep their patients overnight.

The risks primarily relate to infections possible for any surgery, because an implant does necessitate one or more small incisions. Infections are fairly easy to treat but make the penis sore, requiring antibiotic injections or pills for several days. A man cannot use the penis for intercourse for at least two weeks, of course, until the surgeon reexamines him for adequate healing and gives the go-ahead. About 90 percent of men report satisfaction with the results.

There are two types of penile implants. For each, apparatuses are placed into the two upper penile spongy bodies (corpora cavernosa). The first type of implant, flexible rods, has been used the longest. There are no moving parts or complicated mechanisms. They are simply rods that render the penis semierect at all times. They don't shrink in size or become larger. When a man doesn't need his penis for intercourse, he bends it down into place. When he's ready for intercourse, he bends it up. One complaint is, of course, that the erection is always there and potentially discernible. However, loose clothing and padding can hide it.

The other type of implant, the inflatable prosthesis, is more popular. There is a greater risk of infection after surgery and more mechanical failures with this type, though. The prosthesis has two balloonlike devices that the surgeon places into each of the corpora cavernosa. Attached to them is tubing that leads to a pump and a reservoir of liquid, usually sterile water or a saltwater solution similar to natural body fluids. When the man is ready to activate his erection, he locates the manual hydraulic pump the surgeon placed either inside the scrotum or inside the lower abdomen. Using a press and release motion on the skin over the pump, the man inflates the "balloons" in his penis. As they fill, his penis becomes larger and stiffer. When he finishes intercourse, he presses a valve also located under the skin that allows the fluid to drain back into the reservoir.

Both types of penile implants should last many years, but the flexible rod type lasts longer. Since so many men like the results, the number of implant surgeries is increasing. However, don't turn to such a radical solution without carefully examining the causes for your erectile problem and trying first to solve them using less invasive methods.

Vascular surgery.   Several vessels supply blood to the penis, most notably the abdominal aorta, iliac, and internal pudendal arteries. One procedure that may help reestablish blood flow to the penis is an endarterectomy. The surgeon opens the affected artery, removes the blockage, and sews the artery shut again.

Another option is a bypass. Just as a man who has clogged heart vessels may need a coronary bypass operation, so the blood flow to his penis may need to be rerouted around the affected penile artery. This type of bypass operation is not as serious or life-threatening as a coronary bypass, of course, but it is major surgery.

Sometimes, though, the problem isn't that a clogged artery hampers blood flow into the penis. In the course of a complete physical and sexual examination, including penile blood flow studies during erection, the physician discovers excessive blood leakage from the corpora cavernosa or corpus spongiosum into the penile veins. Sometimes surgery can repair these leaks.

There is much to consider when determining the best course

of action for surgically treating erectile dysfunction because these are not minor procedures. Many physicians believe that if surgery is the treatment of choice, a penile implant is safer and has a better success rate for restoring erections than repairing blood vessels. Some men would rather opt for the somewhat riskier vascular surgery to improve blood flow than have something artificial put in the penis that they must "wear" twenty-four hours a day thereafter.

Other factors are expense, insurance coverage, length of recovery, and skill of the surgeon. Ask your family doctor for a recommendation. Investigate how many operations the surgeon has done and with what rate of success. Ask for names of other patients treated who will talk to you about their experiences. It is also perfectly acceptable to travel to a hospital that performs a high volume of the type of operation you want in order to get a more adept surgeon.

No More Excuses

It's amazing how much better we feel psychologically when we learn new tricks to extend our sexual capacity. While I understand the deeply personal nature of sexual problems and the embarrassment of men who finally admit to having one, I assure you that there is hope—tremendous hope!

Don't let yourself hide in shame. The greater shame is in refusing help. The problem won't improve if you just wait. Don't lie to yourself that it doesn't matter anyway. Would you stop eating permanently if you lost your appetite? Of course not. You would find out what was wrong and fix it. Otherwise, you'd starve to death. Then why abandon sex when your libido disappears or your penis doesn't work correctly? To do so is sexual suicide, because you're starving key aspects of being male and being human.

While your sexual worth isn't tied to a functioning penis and there are ways to remain sexually active without an erection, you must first learn all you can about why the problem appeared and how to restore it or maximize your remaining potential. Even if you permanently lose erectile function from a tragedy such as spinal cord injury, though, you can learn how to have orgasms or intercourse in new ways and have a sexually fulfilling marriage. The real test of courage is how bravely you face the problem and ask for help, not how long you hide your unnecessary pain.

5

Pain during Sex

Pain interrupting any enjoyable activity is a disappointing reminder that our aging bodies are betraying us yet again. Sexual pain is especially disturbing because it's also embarrassing, so we tend to let problems related to our sexual organs fester. Pain related to sex rarely disappears without treatment, though. Failure to get help can even lead to permanent damage or sexual dysfunction. Pain is an important signal that something is wrong and that you need help.

Women's Sexual Pain

Pain in the External Genitals

While most sexually related pain women have occurs during intercourse, sometimes it's located in the clitoris or on the labia. Perhaps you need to stop using a spermicidal gel or a cosmetic product that's irritating the genitals. Sometimes soreness of the clitoris and labia is related to inadequate vaginal lubrication. (Moisture from the vagina also reduces friction on the external surfaces during foreplay.) An ingrown pubic hair can cause labial pain. If you've ever had one, you know how difficult it is to extract the hair with tweezers, because you have to use a mirror. Often the best solution is a warm compress and the passage of time. If it becomes infected, see your doctor.

At other times, pain is due to infection. Some nonprescription remedies alleviate inflammation and soreness, such as aloe vera gel or an anesthetic cream made just for the external genitals. However, these products don't treat the underlying infection. It's always wise to see your physician when you suspect a vaginal or vulvar infection, unless you know the symptoms are due to a yeast infection, because you've had one before and the symptoms are the same. In that case you can buy a nonprescription medication—for example, Monistat, Mycelex, or others. These do nothing for vaginitis due to a bacterial, viral, protozoal, or a sexually transmitted infection such as gonorrhea, though.

Sometimes when a postmenopausal woman hasn't had sexual activity for several years (including masturbation), her clitoris becomes "glued" in place under the clitoral hood by adhesions, bands of fibrous connecting tissue. When the clitoris moves during stimulation, the adhesions pull and cause pain. A physician can release them during a pelvic examination using a localized anesthetic.

Pain during Intercourse

Vaginal pain during intercourse—dyspareunia—is serious because it blocks sexual enjoyment and can lead to a sexual dysfunction called vaginismus. If a woman tries to ignore dyspareunia, she will eventually start dreading sex. It can be hard to know which came first, though, lack of desire for intercourse or intercourse pain. A woman may have no interest in sex because she knows intercourse has been hurting, so she's anxious about facing it again. This anxiety inhibits her ability to relax, enjoy foreplay, and become lubricated well. Eventually she tightens up and has spasms in the muscles around the vagina. Therefore, intercourse can hurt for psychological as well as physical reasons. Let's look first at factors that make intercourse hurt because something is wrong physically.

Estrogen deficiency.   The most common cause of dyspareunia in women around the age of or past menopause is vaginal dryness. When the ovaries stop functioning, estrogen drops, bringing changes that include decreased production of vaginal moisture.

Furthermore, the vaginal wall becomes more fragile as the surface lining thins, making it prone to tiny tears and irritation. If you're already on estrogen and still don't have enough vaginal moisture, ask your physician for estrogen cream. Use it on your labia and in your vagina at least three times a week in addition to taking your regular estrogen.

If a woman hasn't yet reached menopause or is already on estrogen therapy but still has vaginal dryness making intercourse uncomfortable, foreplay is probably not lasting long enough before trying to insert the penis. It's possible, too, that foreplay is long enough but that the woman isn't becoming sufficiently aroused due to lack of sexual desire or improper foreplay technique.

Other than estrogen replacement therapy, the best solution for vaginal dryness is to use an artificial lubricant. The cheapest is saliva, but it tends to evaporate quickly and may not be available in sufficient quantities. Other nonprescription choices include suppositories that melt in the vagina, such as Lubrin, or gels and creams, such as Replens, Vagisil, and K-Y. Choose water-soluble lubricants because they don't adhere to tissues as long as oil-soluble lubricants do, making them easier for the body to clear.

Oil-soluble lubricants are acceptable for use on the labia and clitoris, though, because you can wash them off during your next bath with soap and water. The best ones are unscented, to avoid an allergic reaction more likely to occur upon contact with mucous membranes. Acceptable oil-soluble lubricants are mineral oil, unscented baby oil, petroleum jelly, or even oils used for cooking. Stay away from waxy substances, hand lotions, cold creams, or products containing medications (arthritis rubs, antibiotic ointments, hemorrhoid creams, and so forth). Many of these substances contain chemicals that are irritating to mucous membranes. Furthermore, substances are absorbed into the bloodstream more rapidly when applied to mucous membranes instead of dry skin.

Vaginal adhesions. Postmenopausal women who haven't regularly engaged in intercourse can develop vaginal adhesions over the years. These bands of tissue may so extensively obstruct the vagina that intercourse is impossible. Your physician can snip adhesions during a pelvic examination, making the vagina accessible again. Minor bleeding lasts an hour or two, but the procedure is quite painless.

Any woman who hasn't had intercourse for several months or

years would be wise to get a thorough pelvic examination before resuming sexual activity. If she is postmenopausal and hasn't been taking estrogen, she should begin to do so at least a month before resuming intercourse, taking both estrogen pills by mouth and applying estrogen cream to the vagina.

Pelvic inflammatory disease. Pelvic inflammatory disease (PID) is infection and inflammation of internal female organs, particularly the Fallopian tubes and ovaries. Microbes responsible are usually sexually transmitted diseases such as gonorrhea or chlamydia, making it more common in women who don't restrict their sexual partners. Sometimes chronic PID sets in because antibiotics don't destroy all the germs, the woman doesn't seek treatment, or she doesn't finish all her medication, thereby allowing the infection to persist for months or even years. Eventually PID causes infertility due to scarring and blockage of the Fallopian tubes.

A woman with PID often complains of pain with intercourse because thrusting movements of the penis against the cervix cause movement of the uterus, the Fallopian tubes, and even the abdominal organs around them. Even if she reaches orgasms only through clitoral stimulation, the spasms of her uterus during orgasm can still be painful in the presence of PID. Medical treatment is essential.

Vaginal infections. The clinical terms for a vaginal infection are "vaginitis" and "vaginosis." Several microbial agents can cause vaginal pain or unusual secretions. Some germs are sexually transmitted diseases and some are normal microbes that just grow too rapidly. An older woman risks sexually transmitted diseases if she's having extramarital sex, or if her husband is having sex with someone else in addition to her.

However, if you are remaining sexually faithful to each other, then vaginal infections are probably due to overgrowth of germs found normally in the vagina. Overgrowth sometimes comes from taking antibiotics for infections elsewhere in the body that kill normal bacteria in the vagina, too, allowing other microbes there to multiply more rapidly. Sometimes bacteria from the rectal area are inadvertently transferred into the vaginal opening. Other factors promoting vaginitis include stress, anything that makes the normally acid vagina more alkaline, having less resilient vaginal tissues following menopause, or being diabetic. Often, though, it's impossible to determine why vaginitis occurs.

If you have burning, itching, pain, or drainage from your vagina (other than a normal amount of clear mucus), see your physician immediately. Some infections produce a sticky white discharge with a yeasty smell or no odor (yeast infections); a grayish, fishy-smelling discharge (bacterial vaginosis); a yellowish or cloudy liquid (gonorrhea); a frothy, greenish-yellow mucus with a foul odor (trichomonas), and so forth. Delaying treatment doesn't help. Vaginitis rarely goes away on its own, and soon you will be miserable. Symptoms range from mild discomfort to excruciating itching and pain. Sex is out of the question during a flare-up. It can even hurt to urinate, because the urinary opening is sore and urine burns. The vaginal opening, labia, and clitoris itch and burn dreadfully, too.

Stop intercourse until symptoms subside after treatment begins. This keeps you from infecting your husband if the cause is a sexually transmitted disease, and will prevent you from having dyspareunia, causing more tissue irritation, and developing sexual anxiety. In the meantime, satisfy your husband externally, and he can do the same for you *if* you wish.

It's normal for the clitoris to have heightened sensitivity during vaginitis. Because vulvar tissues become inflamed and more reactive, your clitoris may respond rapidly to very delicate stimulation *if* you can bear for it to be touched at all. As treatment begins to work and as symptoms disappear, there comes a point at which sexual stimulation can feel especially good because genital tissues are hypersensitive and just barely "itchy" enough for friction to feel great.

Take all the medicine prescribed, and don't stop when symptoms disappear. Otherwise the strongest germs survive and regrow to cause even worse infections that may not respond to standard medications.

You can prevent most vaginal infections by having monogamous sex, wiping from front to back after bowel movements, eating dairy products with active lactobacillus cultures (yogurt especially), bathing the genitals and rectal area well with soap and water daily, and avoiding douches (especially any that neutralize the acidity of the vagina). Some women swear that installing a bidet or rinsing their genital and rectal areas well with a hand-held shower sprayer greatly reduces the frequency of vaginitis. Also, wear cotton panties to aerate the genitals. Avoid bubble baths. Don't wear clothes tight in the crotch because they trap moisture. You may even need to give up pantyhose temporarily because synthetic fibers prevent evaporation.

> *The first time I had a vaginal infection I waited too long to get help. I'd heard about vaginitis but didn't think I was doing anything to get infected. It started with just a little itchiness around my clitoris, but within a day after that my vagina felt like it was on fire. Jim and I tried to have intercourse, but afterward the opening to my vagina felt like all the skin had been rubbed off. Peeing made me cry. It sounds odd, but the only way I could get relief was to use the shower sprayer on the gentle setting "down there." The cool water relieved some of the pain, and the gentle pressure helped with the itching. My doctor said it was a yeast infection. She told me how to recognize it if I ever got another one, and wrote down the medicine to use. I now know to start using it at the first sign of an infection, but I still can't stand to have sex for two or three days.*

Bladder infection (cystitis). It's rather easy for bacteria to work their way up the short female urinary tube into the bladder. Because the bladder sags with age, the distance becomes even shorter, and infections are more likely. The urinary tube lining also loses resilience as estrogen drops. Pressure on an infected bladder during intercourse may cause pain, but the external urinary opening (meatus) also burns and becomes very sore. The meatus (pronounced "me-ay-tus") sits inside the labia at the top of the vaginal opening, a position that makes it susceptible to friction during intercourse. Sometimes intercourse irritates the meatus, leading to "meatitis," an inflammation that mimics a urinary tract infection.

Any time a woman has burning during urination, an urge to urinate that's hard to control, or finds she is urinating small amounts frequently, she needs immediate help for a possible bladder infection. If untreated, the infection can ascend into and damage the kidneys. Reduce risk of developing a urinary tract infection by wiping from front to back after a bowel movement, drinking enough fluids to keep the bladder washed out, and urinating after sex to rinse out bacteria intercourse may have pushed into the meatus and urinary tube.

> *About four years ago I married for the second time. Though he was forty-eight at the time, Gary is ten years younger than I and has amazing sexual stamina. We went on a cruise for our honeymoon. It was heaven, except for one thing. We had sex so long, hard, and often that I developed a bladder infection. The ship's doctor was very kind and said I had "honeymoon cystitis"—something he saw all the time, being in that line of work. He told me something I've never forgotten: always get up to pee after sex.*

Vaginal fibrocity.   Anything that causes the vaginal lining to toughen renders it less expandable during sexual arousal and intercourse. When tissues do not engorge and expand well, pain can result. Vaginal fibrocity is due to such things as scarring from vaginal surgery, or radiation therapy for cancer in the pelvis. Only by doing a thorough vaginal examination can a physician identify the location causing the pain. He or she may be able to excise or release scar tissue, alleviating sexual discomfort. Sometimes estrogen in the form of vaginal cream helps, too.

Endometriosis.   Endometriosis is a condition only in premenopausal women, in which the uterus lining (endometrium) works its way into the abdomen through the Fallopian tubes. As the monthly hormone cycle passes through the endometrial growth phase, misplaced tissue in the abdomen also grows. The pockets of endometrium also degenerate and bleed during the menstrual period. Since there is no place for this tissue and blood to go, surrounding areas become irritated and painful. During intercourse, especially deep intercourse that jostles internal organs, a woman with endometriosis often has pain.

Treatments include hormonal therapy to control the menstrual cycle, pain relievers, or surgery to remove endometrial tissue. In severe cases that don't respond to conservative therapy, the physician may recommend a hysterectomy (see chapter 6). Menopause ultimately brings relief as menstrual periods cease. During the process of menopause, however, menstrual periods become irregular and more frequent, temporarily worsening endometriosis.

Other causes of painful intercourse.   Other reasons why a woman may experience pain during intercourse include the following, requiring medical intervention:

- uterine fibroids: tissue in the uterus wall that grows into lumps varying in size from microscopic to several inches thick
- abdominal or pelvic ligaments torn during accidents or trauma
- uterine tumors: benign growths or endometrial cancer
- cervical cancer
- uterine prolapse: dropping of the uterus into the vagina because age-weakened ligaments and muscles no longer support its weight
- rectocele: bulging of the rectum into the vagina
- cystocele: protrusion of the bladder into the vagina

Regardless of the cause, if you allow pain to continue without seeing your physician for treatment, you'll begin to fear intercourse and can develop a sexual dysfunction called vaginismus.

Vaginismus

Vaginismus is painful spasming of vaginal muscles so severe that it's difficult to insert the penis into the vagina. Vaginismus in young women is more likely to arise from sexual inhibitions and anxieties that make them tense in anticipation of sex. Vaginismus can also develop later in life when intercourse becomes painful for any reason, particularly if a woman allows the discomfort to continue so long that she starts to dread sex. Any factor that creates anxiety can cause vaginismus and sexual pain.

> *Mack was sixty-seven when he had his first heart attack. He was determined not to let it stop him, though, and bounced back as fast as his doctor would let him. However, I was worried to death. His heart attack gave me such a scare I spent the next six months on pins and needles. Every little twinge he had nearly gave me my own heart attack. He just wouldn't slow down. During sex was the worst. I thought he could die right during intercourse. I couldn't relax enough to get turned on. Sex started to hurt, and I knew exactly why—I was afraid.*

In vaginismus, muscles around the outer third of the vagina involuntarily spasm and squeeze down, including the pubococcygeus (PC) muscles, other muscles encircling the vaginal opening, and even the inner thighs in severe cases. Through no conscious effort, the vagina essentially shuts because of tightly contracting muscles. If the couple attempts intercourse anyway, the woman experiences severe pain.

Sometimes intercourse is impossible because muscles contract so tightly. One reason rape hurts is because these same muscles work as a defense when women feel threatened by unwanted sex. Some also experience vaginismus when anticipating a pelvic examination. Normally a vaginal exam and Pap smear don't hurt, but some women find it so difficult to relax that their bodies fight all the way.

The first step of therapy is to stop intercourse until further notice. You must break the pain and anxiety cycle until you find out what's wrong, give the treatment ample opportunity to work so pain is no longer likely, and feel psychologically ready to try intercourse again. Moving ahead before completing these steps will only cause more pain, reinforcing your fear. You'll probably find that being told to stop having intercourse is a tremendous emotional relief and takes the pressure off while you look for answers. As you work through therapy, though, don't forget that your husband's sexual needs are still important. You can function creatively using oral and manual sex to satisfy him temporarily.

The next step in treatment is a thorough physical and sexual examination to determine any physical reasons for pain during intercourse. However, whether there is a physical cause or your vaginismus is from a psychological anxiety, you must also overcome the response that causes the vaginal muscle spasms. Fixing the physical problem doesn't necessarily cure the vaginismus.

You may need the help of a counselor or a psychologist to help you overcome fears of or guilt about sex. In addition, start practicing the sensate focusing and nondemand pleasuring exercises with your husband described in chapter 3. They will help you become comfortable and relaxed when your husband touches your body, allowing you to enjoy sexual contact again short of intercourse. Since these techniques don't include putting anything into the vagina yet, you can float in the pleasures of external physical love.

While working through these suggestions, practice Kegel exercises to help you control the muscles that spasm during intercourse, because Kegel exercises utilize the PC muscles. To find the PC muscles, start and stop your urine, noting which muscles you use. Tighten and release them as many times and as fast as you can several times a day. Also practice tightening and holding your PC muscles in tension as long as possible. This helps you not only to identify the problem area anatomically, but also gives you practice controlling affected muscles so you can consciously relax them. (It also helps bladder control if you have trouble with urine leakage.)

Once you resume intercourse you may find that doing Kegel exercises repeatedly just before penile insertion fatigues the PC muscles, making them less likely to contract painfully during intercourse. Another technique that counteracts contractions of the PC muscles is to "bear down" during penile insertion, as if you were trying to urinate or have a bowel movement. If you experience a vaginal spasm, don't give up too quickly. Sometimes patience pays off because the muscles fatigue and relax reflexively after a while.

Relaxation techniques may help, too. Before having sex, take a long, hot bath. Think about how much you're going to enjoy being with your husband. Listen to soft music or have a glass of wine. Recall your childbirth classes and use Lamaze breathing techniques during the first minute or two of intercourse. Slow, controlled breathing in through the nose and out through the mouth focuses attention away from pain.

Another treatment for vaginismus involves vaginal dilators, cigar-shaped rods made of plastic or metal. Dilators are about 6 inches long, ranging in size from ¼ inch to 1¼ inches in diameter. Obtain dilators from a physician, sex therapist, or medical supply company. You can even fashion your own from items found around the home, but be sure to thoroughly wash them first; avoid anything coated with a substance that might flake off; use only unbreakable, nontoxic materials; and make sure the tip is rounded and smooth.

Start with the smallest dilator first, inserting it slowly into your vagina with plenty of lubricant, leaving it there for fifteen minutes. Do this at least three or four times a day. Once you can insert the dilator comfortably, masturbate to orgasm with the dilator in place. Then move up to the next size the next day and repeat the process until you can use the largest size.

Now it's time to involve your husband. Many women find that they can insert the dilators alone, but with their husbands present, they again feel anxiety. Therefore, take this as slowly as needed. Don't even use the dilators at first. Start by putting your own hand on your thigh and concentrate just on relaxing that leg. Then let your husband put his hand on your thigh while you continue to relax. When ready, let your husband gently and slowly insert the smallest dilator, using plenty of artificial lubricant and clitoral stimulation. Move on to larger dilators over the next sessions. Practice letting him bring you to a clitorally stimulated orgasm with the dilator in your vagina. Some couples like using the husband's finger instead of a dilator, which is fine, too. He can start by slipping one finger into your vagina, then two at a time, then three at a time.

Once you're comfortable having the largest dilator in your vagina with your husband present, reintroduce intercourse. Again, control the speed at which you progress. Decide how close you'll let his penis get to your vagina, allowing it to come closer over time. Continue deep breathing and relaxation exercises. Your husband is not to make any sudden moves. When ready, let him put his penis next to your vaginal opening, but don't attempt to insert it. Just let it rest there for a session or two.

Only when completely ready for the penis and well lubricated should you then slowly press against it and work it into your vagina. Tell your husband not to do any thrusting yet. Just feel the penis sitting there with no movement. Relax your PC muscles completely and concentrate on pleasurable sensations. Some women find that *intentionally* squeezing the penis with the PC muscles enhances their pleasure. Sometimes women prefer certain intercourse positions for reintroducing the penis to the vagina, such as the one in which the wife straddles her husband while he lies on his back. This makes it easier for her to control the rate of thrusting and the depth of penetration.

Another solution to vaginismus is to let yourself have a clitoral orgasm before trying intercourse. You'll be more likely to be lubricated, you'll feel more relaxed and mellow, and vaginal muscles are less likely to contract because they're tired from spasming during orgasm. Intercourse is often much easier at this point. Whether you use this strategy or not, always have adequately long foreplay, use plenty of artificial lubricant if needed, choose the intercourse position you prefer, and control the rate of penile insertion.

Vaginismus is a common problem most women experience to some degree sometime during their lives. You can overcome it, though, by treating physical reasons for pain during intercourse, examining your attitudes toward sex and their origins, and re-learning how to relax during penile insertion.

SEXUAL PROBLEMS CAUSING PAIN FOR BOTH MEN AND WOMEN

Usually reasons for sexual pain are completely different for men than for women because anatomy and psyches differ so much. The few exceptions, though, have to do with sexually transmitted diseases (STDs). Being older doesn't make you immune to STDs. Extramarital sex opens the door for genital infections of all kinds. Even condoms are little protection against STD viruses, contrary to what you hear in the popular media, because pores in the latex are larger than a virus. Marital fidelity is always the better choice. One situation in which you can contract a genital infection without committing adultery, though, is a herpes outbreak.

Herpes on the genitals originates from sex with someone who has active herpes, or by transferring the virus from a cold sore on the mouth to the genitals. People can even infect their own genitals by unconsciously touching their own cold sores and then their genitals. Another problem is that women with herpes on the cervix cannot see or usually feel an outbreak and may not be aware that they're contagious.

Herpes isn't dangerous except to newborn babies, but is associated with a higher incidence of cervical cancer, so it's important for women with genital herpes to get regular Pap smears. Otherwise it's mostly an annoyance and can hurt, particularly during sex. Many factors can bring on a new outbreak, but some people go for years without one.

There's no cure for herpes. If you get it, you'll always have it. Prescription medications can shorten the duration and severity of each outbreak, though. During an eruption, avoid contact of that site with another person or other parts of your own body. Keep the site clean and dry.

Other STDs can also cause pain during sexual contact, but some are painless at first (such as syphilis sores or HIV, the AIDS virus). All STDs necessitate cessation of sexual activity to prevent spreading the germs until treated (if a cure exists for that particular disease). Whenever you develop a sore on or abnormal discharge from your genitals, immediately abstain from all sexual contact and see your physician—even if you have remained sexually faithful to your partner.

MEN'S SEXUAL PAIN

Most sexual pain in men relates to the prostate, especially as they get older. It can become infected or enlarge to the point where it puts pressure on the urinary tube. Prostate growth is so common that it almost seems normal. Sometimes enlargement is due to cancer, though, a condition that affects sexuality in more ways than just by causing pain. Chapter 7 addresses these problems and more. Therefore let's look instead at other sources of pain related to the male genitalia.

Balanitis

Balanitis, an infection of the foreskin and head of the penis (the "glans"), is usually due to bacteria from the rectal area or poor hygiene. Balanitis rarely occurs in circumcised men because it's easier for them to keep the penis clean. Usually balanitis poses a problem when a man cannot or does not retract his foreskin and wash under it thoroughly regularly. Secretions, urine, and other deposits build up into a sticky white substance called smegma. Smegma is a good growth medium for bacteria. The area underneath the foreskin also promotes bacterial growth because of the dark, moist, warm environment.

Symptoms of balanitis include tenderness, redness, and sometimes a bad odor. During sexual stimulation, when the foreskin normally slips back and forth, friction of the hand or vagina against the penis causes pain. Sufficiently long stimulation to the point of orgasm may be out of the question. Treatment requires antibiotics. In severe cases, circumcision may be necessary.

Most often balanitis occurs in situations where bathing facilities or typical hygiene routines are impossible, such as in combat, on camping trips, and in other circumstances. Any condition that causes an uncircumcised man to lose use of his arms (such as progressive neuromuscular diseases, stroke, or spinal cord injury) makes him dependent on someone else to provide necessary personal hygiene. An older man with Alzheimer's disease may forget to attend to personal cleanliness. In cases like these, too, balanitis becomes a greater risk.

Last summer my son and two grandsons went hiking with me in the mountains for ten days. We were all Boy Scouts from way back and knew about purifying drinking water, hanging food in the trees to keep it from the bears, and carrying all our trash out with us. We knew how to prevent dehydration, treat foot sores, and manage poison ivy. One thing I never learned about or had trouble with before, though, was getting an infection on my penis. Halfway through the trip I started getting sore. When I could finally get some privacy to check myself out, the whole tip was bright red. For those last five days, I was in torture. Every step I took jostled it. I eventually wrapped it up with a bandage from our first-aid kit and took aspirin. Not knowing what was wrong, I had no idea what else to do. When we got back to civilization, for the first time in my life I didn't fight going to the doctor. He said my foreskin had gotten infected from not taking baths on the hike. I couldn't stand for Annette to touch me for two weeks after that. I still go hiking, but now I take along Wet Wipes. I also make sure the triple antibiotic cream is in the first-aid kit.

If you develop balanitis and don't get relief by stepping up your bathing habits and keeping the area under the foreskin dry, try applying an antibiotic ointment and taking a pain reliever. Consult your physician if symptoms persist after two or three days.

Phimosis

Phimosis affects only uncircumcised men. After decades of no difficulty with the foreskin, sometimes for no apparent reason it becomes so tight during erection that it becomes impossible to retract. It restricts blood flow, as if the foreskin were a tourniquet. The only one solution to this painful problem is an emergency circumcision.

Circumcision

Circumcision is more complicated for the adult male than for a baby, whose physician performs it a day or so after birth. If you need a circumcision, you'll probably have a general anesthetic so you will "sleep" during the operation. Removal of the foreskin is not difficult, but can require stitches that must be removed a few days later. Sometimes overnight hospitalization is necessary. Abstain from use of the penis for sexual activity for two to three weeks afterward.

The first time you have an erection after circumcision, the scar tissue at the incision may feel strange. Scar tissue doesn't stretch as well as normal tissue. Some tightness and a tingling sensation are normal, temporary, and usually not of great significance. As time passes, erections gradually stretch the scar and full sensation returns to the incision site. Speak to your physician about any problems.

Penile Fracture

The penis doesn't contain bone, regardless of it being called a "boner" when erect. However, a rare penile problem is similar to a bone breaking. A penile fracture occurs when the shaft of the penis suddenly bends during intercourse, accompanied by a cracking sound, pain in the penis, and immediate loss of erection. The tunica albuginea (the fibrous sheath around the corpora cavernosa) has ruptured. Usually this happens during vigorous, rapid thrusting when the penis comes out of the vagina and doesn't hit the vaginal opening straight upon reentry. Resulting pressure causes the penis to bend abnormally.

> I'd never heard of a penile fracture, but now know firsthand what it is. Well, here's what happened. By the way, you should know that Tina really gets into sex and likes it hard and deep. One time I was on my back and she was on top. She was bouncing high before every thrust and coming down hard. Well, she came down just an inch off target and my penis doubled over about three inches down from the tip like a broken stick. And it sounded like a stick snapping in two. Well, I'm sure you can imagine what that felt like. My penis started getting black and blue in just minutes and hurt like it was broken for sure.

If this happens to you, don't just nurse it alone for a few days in hopes it will feel better again soon. Surgery is often necessary to remove blood that leaked through the tunica albuginea into penile tissues. The corpora cavernosa sometimes need repair, too. Failure to obtain treatment can result in loss of erectile ability, so this certainly isn't a time to believe that time heals all wounds.

Testicular Torsion

Testicular torsion occurs when a testicle twists or turns on the "cord" on which it hangs in the scrotum. Just as the neck of an inflated balloon becomes tight when twisted, so blood vessels to the testicle become tightly constricted during testicular torsion. The constriction reduces blood supply to the testicle. The first symptom is usually pain, then swelling. The only treatment for testicular torsion is emergency surgery. If the surgeon doesn't loosen the constriction and correct the torsion, the testicle will die within a few short hours and shrink over the next few months. It's crucial that you go to an emergency room immediately any time you have pain or abnormal swelling in your scrotum. The safety window is short (four hours maximum), so don't delay. Testicular torsion occurs more often in young men, but happens rarely in older men, too, most often during lively sexual intercourse.

Epididymitis

A more common problem causing scrotal pain in older men is epididymitis, an infection in the epididymis, the portion of the sperm tract that loops over the testicle and leads to the vas deferens (where vasectomies are done). Usually infection starts in the urinary tract, with germs moving backward into the sperm tubing. Symptoms include fever, burning during urination, and gradually increasing scrotal pain and swelling, often made worse by vigorous exercise or sexual activity. Since it can also occur simultaneously with a prostate infection, orgasm may hurt, too. Eventually pain may radiate into the lower abdomen.

Your physician will probably prescribe antibiotics and anti-inflammatory medicine such as aspirin. Treatment involves bed rest for several days and wearing a scrotal support. Avoid strenuous exercise for at least two weeks. Report any sudden pain, since testicular torsion sometimes occurs with epididymitis. Scrotal tenderness may persist for several weeks.

Sexual activity is permitted, but avoid positions that let the scrotum dangle. It would be better to let your wife be on top and to support your scrotum underneath with a small rolled-up towel. If sex is too painful, temporarily discontinue intercourse. Help your wife to meet her sexual needs through clitoral stimulation until you recover.

Priapism

Priapism is unwanted, prolonged erection. In mild episodes, the erection lasts an hour beyond orgasm or after sexual stimulation ceases. Severe cases of untreated priapism have lasted days. This painful problem is not always associated with sexual activity, though, and may occur spontaneously in certain medical conditions.

Causes of priapism include medications injected into the penis to bring on an erection, some blood pressure medicines, nerve damage to the spinal cord, and blood disorders (e.g., sickle cell anemia) that cause red blood cells to clump and block small vessels draining blood from the penis. Regardless of why priapism starts, you need immediate treatment any time your erection lasts an hour longer than you want it to. Delaying can damage the corpora cavernosa and cause permanent erectile dysfunction.

While you wait at home the first hour to see if the erection will subside by itself, drink three glasses of water or other liquid as fast as you can to dilute the blood and dislodge clumped cells. Apply an ice pack to your penis. If you have a prescription for an antianxiety medication, take a pill. If not, drink a glass of wine or other alcoholic beverage. Some men find that a warm enema does the trick.

If none of these ideas helps, see your physician right away. You may get an intravenous line (IV) for fluids to dilute your blood, or blood vessel dilators, muscles relaxants, or other medications may be administered. If you have sickle cell anemia or another blood-clumping problem, an exchange transfusion of blood can help. As a last resort, surgery can divert blood away from your penis or out of the corpora cavernosa into the corpus spongiosum. Generally these operations don't cause permanent erectile problems, although you may need reparative work later.

Other Conditions

Many other problems men can suffer that cause pain during sexual activity include:

- hydrocele: collection of fluid in the outermost covering of the testes
- varicocele: a varicose vein in the scrotum
- testicular trauma: injury to the scrotum from a blow or a puncture
- hernia: protrusion of part of the intestine into the scrotum through a weakened portion of the abdomen's muscular wall

Whenever you notice swelling or pain in the genital or pelvic area, see your physician immediately. Discontinue sexual activity until you receive the "go-ahead."

DON'T WAIT TO GET HELP

There's nothing admirable about tolerating unnecessary pain, especially when the underlying problem can be serious. Shyness or embarrassment you feel about sexual pain is not shared by the professionals who can help. Your problem is no more remarkable to them than broken bones, stomach ulcers, or headaches. They're accustomed to dealing with private and intimate issues. Swallow your feelings and just say the words "It hurts when I have sex." You'll be glad you didn't wait any longer.

6

SEX AFTER A HYSTERECTOMY

In my early days just out of nursing school, I worked in the gynecologic surgery unit of a major hospital. Many of the women we cared for were there for a "hysterectomy with bilateral salpingo-oophorectomy." They were surprisingly stoic in the face of what must have been one of the most frightening ordeals they'd ever encountered. We expertly prevented infections, treated pain, and helped them regain their strength, but neglected one of their biggest concerns: sexuality.

If your nurses and doctors say nothing about sex after your hysterectomy, their silence doesn't mean your sex life is now extinct. That's absolutely *not* true. Nothing taken out during a hysterectomy takes out the ability to have fantastic orgasms. A hysterectomy need be nothing more than a pothole on the road of sexual happiness. The key factor determining your future sexual satisfaction will be whether you learn about your body and adjust to the changes a hysterectomy brings.

WHAT IS A HYSTERECTOMY?

A hysterectomy is surgical removal of the uterus (the womb). It is the most common major surgical operation in the United States.

According to the National Institutes of Health, there are almost seven hundred thousand hysterectomies every year, performed at an average age of forty-three years. American physicians now usually remove the cervix, the lower portion of the uterus that sits down into the vagina, although in years past they left it intact to avoid surgical intrusion into the vagina. European surgeons more often leave the cervix, believing it helps support the upper vagina and avoids sexual nerve damage. If you still have your cervix after a hysterectomy, continue to get Pap smears regularly to screen for cervical cancer.

"Oophorectomy" (pronounce the "oo" as in the word "food") means removal of one ovary or both ovaries. A "bilateral salpingo-oophorectomy" involves removal of both ovaries and Fallopian tubes. Surgeons routinely performed this procedure as part of hysterectomies through the 1970s, and continue to keep it as an option. Even if you're already past menopause, an oophorectomy can diminish your sex drive. Nevertheless, for medical reasons an oophorectomy may sometimes be worthwhile.

A few books available to help you decide whether a hysterectomy is necessary have a decided bias against the surgery. Sometimes, though, a hysterectomy is the best solution to certain problems, such as long-term endometriosis that hasn't responded well enough to other therapies and is so painful it interferes with normal life. (See chapter 5.) Be sure first to investigate thoroughly other options now available that may work as well as a hysterectomy, though, such as embolization to cut blood supply to small fibroids, a myomectomy to remove the uterine lining, endometrial ablation, uterotomy, and so forth. Never resort to a hysterectomy unless it truly is your last choice, because there can be many physical and emotional consequences. And *never* let anyone take your ovaries out unless you have ovarian cancer or such severe problems caused by your ovaries that you've lost all interest in sex anyway.

One valid reason for a hysterectomy may be to remove large fibroids causing persistent bleeding. Fibroids are knots of uterine wall tissue varying from microscopic to several inches thick. Cancer of the uterus, cervix, or ovaries definitely requires a hysterectomy, as does uterine prolapse (bulging of the uterus into or even out of the vagina) that other techniques haven't helped treat. In these cases a hysterectomy provides tremendous relief and improves the quality and extends the length of a woman's life.

I had tried everything: antibiotics, a laparoscopy to burn out the pockets of bleeding tissue in my abdomen, hormone treatments, heating pads and ice packs, every pain reliever from aspirin to Demerol, herbal remedies, exercise, everything I could think of or read about! Some of the treatments helped for a while, but always the pain would return. My abdomen hurt so bad during flare-ups of endometriosis that I was in tears. I couldn't stand to have anyone touch me, let alone try sex. Even when the pain wasn't bad, intercourse hurt whenever my husband shoved his penis around enough to get his climax. Hysterectomy was a big relief. It was the smartest thing I ever did. I only wish I hadn't waited so long!

Before consenting to a hysterectomy, though, get a second opinion and read, read, read! Except in the case of cancer, there is usually time to try medications and other procedures to relieve problems. Ask questions: "If I wait and try other treatments, what risks am I taking? Will I eventually need a hysterectomy anyway? Is it possible or safe for me to become pregnant in the meantime?"

Once the decision is made to proceed, the surgeon will perform the hysterectomy via one of three primary routes: (1) through an abdominal incision about four to six inches long, either vertically between the belly button and the pubic hair or horizontally low on the abdomen (a "bikini" cut); (2) through the vagina, leaving no visible scar; or (3) through a small hole in the front of the abdomen made for a scope, making visualization and removal of the uterus possible. Ovary removal requires the first route.

Before entering the hospital for a hysterectomy you will probably have blood tests, a physical examination, an electrocardiogram (EKG), and perhaps X rays. Early on the morning of the surgery, you'll undergo preoperative "preps" at the hospital. Preps include shaving the skin around the surgical area, a douche, medications to make you drowsy, and perhaps an enema.

By the time I was finally through all the preliminaries before my hysterectomy, I already felt traumatized. Thank God for that shot I got before I went into the operating room. It helped tremendously. I felt as if I was floating and sleepy and that nothing mattered anymore.

The surgery usually lasts one to two hours. Most women receive general anesthesia, although a few undergo the surgery with a spinal anesthetic and remain awake. You'll probably be allowed to sit up and stand briefly later that evening. Your physician may place a tube ("Foley catheter") into your bladder to drain urine over the first night after surgery. Your vagina will remain packed with gauze for a day or two. Most women can go home in two to three days.

CRAZY THINGS YOU MAY HAVE HEARD ABOUT HYSTERECTOMIES THAT ARE NOT TRUE

One of the more vicious tales going around is that the surgeon removes the vagina or sews it shut as part of a hysterectomy, implying that sexual intercourse becomes impossible. The truth is, the surgeon does have to close the vagina to create a dead end where the uterus used to sit, but that place is at the far end deep inside the vagina, not at the outer opening. A few women complain that their hysterectomies left their vaginas a bit shorter, preventing very deep penile penetration, but even then intercourse is still possible.

Another common misconception defies logic. Some women are surprised to learn that after a hysterectomy they will no longer have menstrual periods. Menstruation ceases because the uterus is the source of the menstrual discharge. With no uterine lining to shed, there are no more periods.

Some women mistakenly believe the uterus is essential for orgasms. While the uterus may contract rhythmically during orgasm, it is stimulation of the clitoris, not the uterus, that brings about orgasm. Without the uterus, orgasm continues to be just as pleasurable. (On the other hand, deep intercourse may feel a bit different without a uterus, especially if the surgeon removed the cervix, because the bumping of the penis on the cervix formerly moved the uterus a bit. This movement feels good to some women but is painful to others. Therefore, a few women will miss uterine movement during penile thrusting, but to others it is a big relief.)

Another myth is that removal of the uterus weakens women—that the uterus is a source of strength or power.

> *I knew the surgery would leave me weak for a couple of months,*
> *but more than that, I just knew that without my uterus I wouldn't*

*have the endurance I used to have. I expected trouble keeping up
with the housework and meeting my family's needs.*

The uterus is indeed primarily made of muscle, but it's not a
muscle related to strength or stamina. The uterine muscle performs one job only: pushing a baby out during labor and delivery.

A less common myth is that the uterus rids the body of wastes.
Menstruation is a process of passing unneeded uterine lining tissue, but without the uterus there's no need for menstruation.
Blood lost during menstruation isn't "bad" or old blood the body
needs to eject, as some think.

In spite of endless complaints about menstrual periods, they
do give a certain rhythmic predictability to life. Some women actually grieve cessation of menstruation. They view periods as
signs that all is right with their bodies. It's true that a late menstrual period may indicate anything from pregnancy to hormonal
imbalances to malnutrition to stress, but the actual event of men-
struating is not essential for good health.

Finally, a common myth is that hysterectomies cause weight
gain. The uterus has no relationship to metabolism, though. It's
not a source of vitality or energy. It has no relationship to fat.

HOW A HYSTERECTOMY AFFECTS A
WOMAN'S SEXUAL FEELINGS

Any surgery can leave you feeling powerless, frightened, and violated, but a hysterectomy also affects body image and feelings of
femininity. How you perceive your body in turn affects how you
function sexually. A woman whose life's work has primarily been
the bearing and rearing of children may feel a shift in identity or
purpose in life.

> *After my hysterectomy, I just couldn't stop crying. I felt so silly be-
> cause I'd already gone through the change [menopause] and
> couldn't have babies anymore anyway. But to lose my uterus just
> made it feel so* final! *I couldn't explain my feelings to anyone for
> a long time.*

Having a uterus is proof for many women that they are indeed
female. Without it they may feel as though they've been neutered.

The fact is, though, that gender is not determined by what organs we have. A woman who loses a breast to cancer is no less a woman. A man who has his prostate removed is no less a man. Unfortunately, it's easier to change our bodies with surgery than it is to change our psyches to redefine our self-images after surgery. Long after the incision heals, the mind continues to adjust.

If you've based your female identity on having an intact uterus or ovaries, you must give yourself permission to redefine who you are as a woman. It's much healthier psychologically for all women to characterize their femininity in terms that do not change, such as their worth as women, their personalities, their sense of caring and nurturing, their accomplishments, the fact that their genes will always be coded female, their brains will remain imprinted as female, they have been socialized into the female role, and other lasting elements.

Most women feel some sorrow as they face a hysterectomy, even if it comes as a welcome relief. For younger women, the surgery terminates their ability to bear children. Older women may interpret it as a sign of their aging bodies betraying them. For all women, loss of any body part is traumatic. Loss of a uniquely female body part such as a uterus or ovaries or a breast causes special personal pain.

During the first month after surgery, you'll probably be emotionally unstable. You'll feel sad (even depressed), restless, crabby, and weepy. You'll probably lose your appetite temporarily, a side effect of many major surgeries. Sometimes irritability is due to surgical pain, intestinal gas, or constipation from changes in eating and exercise habits. Sometimes you won't be able to pinpoint the cause. (Some women mistakenly blame emotional changes on the hysterectomy, when in fact they had an oophorectomy and it's the sudden hormonal starvation that is responsible.)

> *For several days, I was a wreck. There just hadn't been much time between when I was told a hysterectomy was my only option and when I had it done. Afterward, I kept shifting between "What have I done?" and "I had no choice." I eventually accepted the necessity of the surgery and worked through the shock and loss, but it took time. Even then, I still found myself crying over the stupidest little things unrelated to the surgery. Thank God, Max hung in there with me through it all. After about five weeks, I returned to my old self.*

Such feelings are normal for a time. Continued or deepening depression requiring medication and professional counseling is not common, though. If your feelings of sadness continue for more than two months or keep you from living a useful, satisfying life, get professional help.

A woman who claims her hysterectomy was "a breeze" is probably hiding her feelings. Physical recovery from major surgery is not only painful physically, but psychologically as well. By denying that removal of her uterus (and possibly ovaries) has any impact, she prevents herself from dealing with fears, going through the healthy stages of grieving, and planning ways to adjust. Blind optimism is often a tool that "brave" women use to preserve their strong image. It can help for another woman who's had a hysterectomy to share her feelings about her own surgery. This breaks through the feelings of aloneness, making expression of true emotions easier.

You might discover that your health caregivers seem insensitive to the significance of a hysterectomy. Perhaps they're encouraging you to have a positive outlook. Perhaps it's because hysterectomies are so common, they seem routine. However, husbands and other loved ones may seem nonchalant on the surface for other reasons. They may be hiding their fears. Any major surgery is not without risk and bluntly reminds them how vulnerable we all are.

The words a woman uses are clues to feelings she's hiding. I often heard women talking about their hysterectomies on the telephone from their hospital beds. Such statements as "They took everything out" were not uncommon. This told me that, even though I well knew there was no way the surgeon took "everything" out, these women were feeling an emotional emptiness and great loss. Some women visualized an empty space where the uterus used to be, not knowing that organs around the site shift to fill that space. Since the uterus is usually smaller than a fist, the abdomen shrinks so little it may look the same size after surgery.

Another common description my patients used was "They cleaned me out." This was disturbing because that implied the uterus and the ovaries were somehow dirty.

I feel like a chicken that's been killed on the farm, sliced open, and all the guts washed out—only they sewed me back up and I'm still alive. It all seems so inhumane somehow.

The sense of being dirty and washed out is especially common for women who have hysterectomies for cancer. The impression of "being diseased" is so devastatingly repugnant to some people's self-image that they psychologically distance themselves from the cancer. After surgery they then feel "cleaned out" both in the sense that the surgeon excised much tissue and because the "dirty" cancer was removed.

THE IMPACT OF HYSTERECTOMY ON THE MARRIAGE

No rule says that if a marriage is weak, a hysterectomy will destroy it. Couples who've learned how to cling together during a crisis instead of withdrawing will find that a hysterectomy is not likely to alienate them, though. On the other hand, a relationship built on superficial attractions and false images makes a woman doubt whether she is still appealing to her husband. Even if she can accept the loss of her uterus, there may be a surgical scar that leaves her feeling ugly. (Fortunately, six months after surgery the scar will probably be just a thin line.) She needs repeated assurance of her husband's unfailing love and acceptance regardless of what happens. She needs to feel that she is still sexy and attractive. Sometimes, though, men have misconceptions, too. If a husband perceives his wife differently after a hysterectomy, he, too, needs education and counseling.

Key to reestablishing your sex life is your attitude about yourself. If you act sexy and show interest in sexual activity, your husband will most likely respond to your lead. His action will be a *reaction* to your behavior. It's a rare husband who can generate enough romance and persuasion to turn around his wife's negative feelings entirely by himself. You must make a serious effort, explaining to him how your sexual needs may have changed. Usually a husband's feelings toward his wife don't change, but he worries about hurting her during sexual intercourse.

> *Betty had always been very healthy. She jogged every other day and was in great shape. When I heard that she was going to need a hysterectomy, I at first thought "No big deal." It came as such a shock to me when I was allowed to see her right after the surgery when she first woke up. She looked very pale, could barely speak, and couldn't even raise up to take a drink of water. I had never seen her like that before. That was when the seriousness of what*

had happened began to hit me. Over the next several weeks, she regained most of her strength and started to return to normal. When we tried to start having sex again, though, I found myself just thinking about whether I was hurting her. Was I putting too much pressure on her tummy? Was my penis pushing in too far? Was I being selfish even wanting sex? All these questions took their toll on me, and I actually had trouble getting an erection for a few weeks until we were finally able to talk it out and I began to relax.

If her husband doesn't express his concerns, a woman may misinterpret his silence or tentative approach as a sign of disinterest or even disgust. As hard as it is to say the words out loud, you'll benefit greatly by opening up to each other, exploring your feelings, and clarifying your needs.

Ask your husband to come with you to at least one doctor's appointment to discuss your fears with a professional together. He should also hear the postoperative instructions given before you leave the hospital. Nurses and doctors can assure him that sexual intercourse will not break open the incision or cause damage once tissues heal in a few weeks.

How a Hysterectomy Changes Sex

Hormones

A hysterectomy removing only the uterus has no impact on hormones. Excision of the ovaries definitely does, though. For that reason many surgeons try to leave at least a portion of one ovary if possible.

We worry first about the impact ovary removal has on estrogen. By taking out both ovaries, a premenopausal woman suddenly enters "surgical menopause." Unless she immediately begins estrogen replacement medication, she'll start showing the signs and symptoms of menopause: hot flashes, vaginal dryness, osteoporosis, acceleration of heart disease risks, shrinking of vaginal tissues, emotional swings, and other problems. Sometimes these symptoms affect women much more profoundly after oophorectomy than during menopause because the drop in hormones is sudden, not allowing adjustment over the span of several years.

Our mothers and grandmothers lived the remainder of their lives without the benefit of estrogen because of physicians' unfounded fears that it caused cancer. However, the problems caused by estrogen deficiency, such as osteoporosis and increased cardiac disease, produce much more illness and death than any of the side effects of estrogen replacement therapy.

Estrogen is not the only hormone lost with ovary removal, however. Testosterone, an important factor in sex drive, also drops. In both men and women, hormones called "androgens" trigger sexual desire. Testosterone is the primary androgen. An abnormally high amount of testosterone in the bloodstream doesn't turn a person into a sex maniac, but having even a little is the best aphrodisiac known. It works in women both by increasing sexual desire and by enhancing response to sexual stimulation.

Ovaries are the major source of androgens. Even after menopause, when estrogen production shuts down, the ovaries continue to make androgens, promoting sexual desire into old age. This is why it's important to keep your ovaries, even if you're past menopause.

> *After my hysterectomy I just wasn't as interested in sex. At first I thought it was because I felt so tired after the surgery. I was so weak that for a month all I wanted to do was sleep. Eventually, though, everything began to return to normal, except for my sex drive. Bob was very patient and tried to understand, but it began to be a sore point between us. At my six-month checkup, I mentioned the problem to my gynecologist. He said I was probably depressed about losing my female organs, and loss of interest in sex was a sign of depression. He prescribed some Prozac, but that didn't help my sex drive at all. I just felt there had to be more to it. I didn't think I was depressed. My hysterectomy had actually been a relief in many ways.*

Unfortunately, some physicians downplay the need for female androgens. They rationalize it by saying that the adrenal glands continue to make small amounts of androgens, but the testimonials of women who disagree are backed by animal studies showing that after ovary removal females display sexual interest less often and rarely initiate sexual contact.

Why not just give a woman a testosterone pill along with her estrogen? Unfortunately, there's no satisfactory way of replacing ovarian androgens. Digestion breaks down testosterone, leaving it virtually useless. Synthetic testosterone in pill form doesn't yield results as good as four other alternatives: testosterone injections, pills that dissolve under the tongue, creams absorbed through the skin, and taking no testosterone at all. Administering testosterone to a woman can cause side effects: increased acne, breast size reduction, facial hair growth, voice deepening, and other male characteristics. If you still want to try testosterone, though, find a physician knowledgeable about replacement of female androgens.

There is hope if you choose not to take testosterone-type medicines, though—if you are willing to take action. The sex drive in humans is different from that in animals because it doesn't rely exclusively on hormones or instinct. Touch, sound, smell, sight, and thought also stimulate the libido. Unlike their animal counterparts, human females don't rely on hormonal estrus ("going into heat") to be interested in sex. Because of this blessing, women can use the triggers of touch, sound, smell, sight, and thought to psychologically build sexual desire leading to sexual arousal, in spite of a drop in testosterone after oophorectomy.

How exactly can you stimulate your sex drive? First, prepare yourself for sex by opening your mind to sexual stimuli. Read an erotic novel. Take a sensuous bath. Fantasize about sex. Use perfume and sexy lingerie, and try other mood-setting techniques. Second, teach your husband how to build your desire through romance, erotic visual images, massage, application of lubricants to your genitals, and so forth, but above all by providing sufficiently long foreplay involving the clitoris. These techniques work much better than fad aphrodisiacs such as herbal preparations.

In light of the problems caused by oophorectomy, the obvious question is "Why ever remove the ovaries?" Some surgeons believe it prevents ovarian cancer. That argument is true, but removal of any body part because something *might* happen is highly questionable. Only if you're at great risk for ovarian cancer should you consider an oophorectomy as a preventive measure. Remember, estrogen replacement therapy will still be important because more women die from complications of osteoporosis than of ovarian cancer.

Better reasons for an oophorectomy include noncancerous ovarian cysts or tumors that are growing and may be painful. In women who had a hysterectomy for endometriosis, endometriosis still can return and become a greater problem, as long as the ovaries continue their monthly hormone production cycles. Other problems worthy of an oophorectomy include scarring of the ovaries or protracted pelvic inflammatory disease (PID) that antibiotics don't cure. If the ovaries cause such severe problems that a woman has lost interest in sex anyway because of pain or other factors, the answer is obvious: oophorectomy.

Changes in a Woman's Anatomy

Not only can ovary removal alter your hormone levels, but also the structure of your internal anatomy changes with any type of hysterectomy. The tenting effect (see chapter 2) disappears during sexual arousal, of course, because the uterus is gone. Most women don't notice any difference, but some miss the passionate desire for penile penetration it creates. You can enhance the urge for intercourse by squeezing the penis with the pubococcygeus (PC) muscles (see instructions on how to do this in chapter 5).

If you neglect to start estrogen medication after oophorectomy, your vagina will thin and become more fragile. Natural lubrication inside the vagina will diminish, even during sexual arousal, making intercourse painful unless you use an artificial lubricant. Without adequate lubrication it's possible for penile thrusting to abrade the vaginal wall, causing even more pain and risking infection.

Sexual Problems

When intercourse hurts, a woman becomes tense in anticipation of the pain, leading to a sexual problem called "vaginismus." Some couples give up on intercourse altogether because of their frustration over vaginismus. (See chapter 5 for help.) Prolonged abstinence from intercourse, especially by women past menopause (whether brought on "surgically" or naturally), causes further shrinkage of vaginal tissues. Eventually some even develop adhesions in the vagina. If they try to begin having intercourse again, they find the vagina has become partially obstructed by the adhesions, requiring minor surgery to release them. Here the old adage "If you don't use it, you'll lose it" holds special meaning.

Put the vagina to the good purpose for which it was designed. Sexual arousal and intercourse are beneficial by improving circulation to the area and bringing more oxygen and nutrition to fragile tissues. Sexual activity stretches and massages your vagina. Lubrication keeps the tissues moist and less susceptible to infections.

Even premenopausal women whose ovaries are intact and

who still have ample estrogen may experience sexual problems after a hysterectomy from fear of pain during intercourse. Any woman can have doubts about her "durability"—her hardiness both for the physical exertion of intercourse and for her surgically traumatized pelvic organs. Expect your abdomen to be tender for at least twelve weeks after the operation, especially if the surgeon made the incision through your abdomen instead of your vagina. The first time you have intercourse, some anxiety wondering what it will feel like is normal. Your husband may worry, too, not wanting to hurt you or damage your incision. If you ignore his fears and show pain or tension, he may develop sexual difficulties, too.

If a hysterectomy involves removal of the cervix, the vagina may be slightly shorter following surgery. Discuss how much shorter with your surgeon before the operation. There may be a good reason for removal of the innermost portion of the vagina, such as cervical cancer. Most women say that any difference in vaginal length has caused no problems with intercourse for them. Certainly you'll want to take intercourse slowly the first few times after surgery and experiment to find a comfortable depth for penile penetration. Postpone vigorous, deep thrusting for at least three months.

Another problem a few women have is decreased vaginal sensation after surgery that included removal of the cervix. Vaginal numbness may result from nerve damage occurring when tissues around the cervix were cut. Unfortunately, numbness that persists for more than three or four months after surgery is likely to be permanent. Intercourse becomes less of a physical pleasure than a psychological one. Fortunately, clitoral sensation is not impaired, and becomes even more critical for sexual satisfaction.

STARTING TO HAVE SEX AGAIN

Wait at least six weeks after a hysterectomy before starting intercourse. The incision has usually healed enough by this time, reducing risks of infection or tearing. Furthermore, at your follow-up examination about four to six weeks after the surgery your physician can assure you if everything is proceeding normally. Occasionally, especially after a vaginal hysterectomy, internal healing takes a little longer.

You needn't wait six weeks to begin any sexual activity, though. Explore other satisfying forms of sexual expression. As soon as ten days after surgery, feel free to stimulate your clitoris to orgasm. During masturbation you can take your time, pay attention to any new sensations, and rebuild confidence in your ability to have an orgasm.

Cuddling and other displays of affection between you and your husband should never have stopped. When hospitalized for any reason, don't let the strangeness of the hospital environment stop physical contact with your husband. While *sexual* contact can wait, closeness through hugs, snuggling in bed together, holding hands, kissing, giving back rubs, and other displays of support and affection will help keep the romance and sexual undercurrent alive.

About two weeks after surgery you can resume more sexually focused activities together. Mutual manual stimulation to orgasm, oral stimulation of each other's genitals, and other techniques that avoid inserting anything into the vagina are good ways to relieve sexual tension and draw closer together during the recovery period. You will tire easily, so choose positions and activities that conserve your energy. If you have an abdominal scar and are self-conscious about it, cover it with sexy lingerie, such as a garter belt, a long camisole, or crotchless panties until you feel more comfortable about your body.

> *It's really ironic that something I had been dreading—a hysterectomy—actually improved our sex life so much. It wasn't the way it improved my health, it was the fact that while I was still healing we had to resort to nontraditional sexual techniques. We explored oral sex for the first time and found it to be utterly delightful! More than delightful—absolutely intense and passionate!*

Once you do resume intercourse, expect mild pain or tenderness for three months or so. Experiment with intercourse positions that avoid pressure on your abdomen or that cause pain. Don't let mild discomfort prevent resumption of sexual activities, however. The anxieties of having major surgery, fears about the risks, interruptions in normal routines, the financial impact, and other problems cause enough marital tension without adding to your stress by abstaining from sex for too long. Sexual intimacy restores the cozy companionship of a good marriage, making other problems easier to solve together.

A few women notice that uterine contractions are absent during orgasm. Orgasms should still feel wonderful, though. Missing uterine spasms is rarely a big concern and doesn't lead to sexual dysfunction.

THE GOOD NEWS ABOUT HYSTERECTOMIES

In spite of the probability that sexual function will change some, most women report that their sex lives don't lose quality after a hysterectomy. In fact, many agree that they enjoy sex more than before the surgery once they get past the three-month recovery period. There are many explanations for the better sex: relief from symptoms or disease that made the hysterectomy necessary; drawing together of the couple as they survive a crisis; freedom from fear of pain, pregnancy, cancer, or the unknown; new confidence from overcoming a difficult challenge; or many other possible personal factors.

> *I found that my hysterectomy was very liberating! Having a hysterectomy was one of the most intelligent things I ever did. Not until it was all behind me did I realize how much anxiety I had felt from abdominal pain. And it was a real pain in the neck, too—but a different kind of pain, the kind that comes from having to haul Kotex around in my purse everywhere I went because I never knew when I would start bleeding again. My mood has improved. I'm not as crabby anymore because I feel better. And sex is great! It doesn't hurt and we can have it anytime we want because I'm never on a "period" anymore.*

Of course, allow yourself time to grieve your loss, too. Losing a uterus (and possibly ovaries) is a major event. The stiff-upper-lip attitude isn't always helpful. People who can help you can't easily break through a wall of cheerfulness or grim determination. Grieving is a healthy, normal process that you should permit and express. Talk to your nurses and doctors about your feelings. Talk to other women who've had hysterectomies. If you have access to the Internet, join a chat room on the subject of hysterectomy.

You can adjust to every alteration in sexual functioning with the right information, an open mind, and a willingness to experiment and change. By taking an active role in recovery and adaptation to life after surgery, you can keep what are usually minor inconveniences from becoming major sexual dysfunctions or possibly even the epitaph of your sex life entirely.

7

Sex and the Prostate

My introduction to prostate problems came between my junior and senior years of nursing school. To earn a little money I took a job for the summer on the night shift as a nursing assistant on the urology floor of a large hospital. Most men were there to get their prostates "reamed out," as the surgeons called it. My duties included irrigating urinary catheters after surgery to keep blood clots from clogging up the tubing and rousting awake men on the mornings of their operations to give them enemas.

My other patients were there for prostate removal to treat cancer. These men were usually tight-lipped about their conditions. Occasionally, though, one would have trouble sleeping, put his light on to make a minor request, and want to talk. Sometimes he just seemed to want company, but it would become apparent he needed a female stranger to reassure him he had made the right decision and that if he lost erectile function after surgery women would still want him.

The year was 1975, though, and there was little hope to offer. Some men cried, most were stoic, and a few even changed their minds and went home without the surgery. I wish I could go back in time to tell those men what I know now about preserving sexual function and staying orgasmic. I wish we then had the courageous examples of other men who have publicly faced prostate cancer, such as Bob Dole, Harry Blackmun, Len Dawson, Johnny Unitas, Richard Bloch, Louis Farrakhan, Eddie Arcaro, Stan Musial, Richard Petty, Ed Asner, Frank Borman, Sidney Poitier, Merv Griffin, Harry Belafonte, Jerry Lewis, Louis Gosset, Jr., Sean Connery, Norman Schwarzkopf, Robert Goulet, Arnold Palmer, Bobby Riggs, and Telly Savalas.

What Is the Prostate?

The prostate gland is a uniquely male organ that exists solely to make most of the ejaculate fluid. This little organ certainly isn't what most men consider to be the central icon of their masculinity. However, it can present challenges to even the most manly person with its embarrassing and annoying interruptions of normal urine drainage. Since the prostate is also part of the reproductive system, sexual implications can become troublesome.

The prostate gland sits just underneath the bladder, where the sperm system joins with the urine system to form the urethra (the passageway through which both urine and ejaculation pass to the outside through the penis). The prostate is normally about 1 inch to 1¼ inches in diameter and roughly globular, shaped like a small turnip. Normally its consistency is firm but slightly spongy.

Because nerve fibers that supply the prostate also come close to nerves supplying organs in the lower abdomen, sometimes prostate pain shows up in the back, the perineum (the area behind the scrotum), the lower abdomen, the testes, or the penis. Unless you know about "referred" pain, you may not realize your prostate is the culprit. An easier symptom to recognize occurs during ejaculation because when the prostate contracts, the spasms of orgasm can hurt. Problems with urination also signal that something is wrong with your prostate.

The challenge then becomes determining what is wrong. Some men claim that certain foods irritate their prostates, or you could have a prostate infection. Perhaps your prostate pain comes from a narrowing of your urinary tube because your prostate has become larger over the years. It's possible you have prostate cancer. Prostate pain can even be psychological in origin, although this isn't likely. Regardless of the cause, your prostate problems can affect sexual enjoyment.

PROSTATITIS

Prostatitis is a condition in which the prostate gland becomes inflamed from some irritant, usually an infection. Bacteria from the rectum or sexual contact with the wife's anal area can cause infections of the prostate. The most common bacteria responsible are *E. coli, Pseudomonas, Proteus,* or *Klebsiella*. Differentiating an infection from other causes of prostatitis can be tricky because the prostate is a difficult organ from which to extract a satisfactory fluid sample for laboratory analysis. It is full of tiny pockets called acini, which hold prostatic fluid. An ejaculation specimen is not always acceptable for diagnosis of infection because the fluid from the prostate becomes diluted with secretions from the testes, the epididymis, Cowper's glands (bulbourethral glands), Littre's glands (periurethral glands), and the seminal vesicles.

For many years physicians couldn't diagnose some types of bacterial infections, and just told a man his prostate was getting old and he was going to have to endure the discomfort. Some physicians called this chronic condition "nonbacterial prostatitis" or "prostatodynia" because they couldn't find the bacteria. Many indiscriminately prescribed newer antibiotics that kill a broader range of bacteria for any noncancerous prostate condition, assuming they were being safe rather than sorry by going ahead with the medication. The problem was, though, as we also discovered from overtreating sore throats and other infections, that the germs mutated. Many have become resistant to the new antibiotics. Antibiotics do not move from the bloodstream into the acini very easily anyway.

Symptoms of Prostatitis

If you've ever had a case of rapid-onset bacterial prostatitis, you know the intense symptoms: painful urination, possibly losing control of your urine, the urge to urinate even when your bladder is empty, and having to get up at night to use the bathroom. The symptoms mimic a bladder infection, which may also coexist with prostatitis.

> *My prostate infection hit me like a truck. Over a period of about six hours, I moved from running a little fever to feeling like someone was sticking a knife up my pee tube. I could hardly bear to pee and tried not to go very often, but soon it felt like I needed to go constantly.*

I drank as little as I could get by with to keep from having to go so much. By the next morning I just couldn't take it anymore and called my doctor's office and demanded an appointment. He put me on antibiotics and by the next day I was feeling much better.

Usually a prostate infection doesn't start rapidly, though. A man with chronic bacterial prostatitis may not even know of his problem unless, in addition to the urinary symptoms, he has pain in the lower back and perineum, a fever, chills, and exhaustion. He probably has pain in his prostate, back, or lower abdomen during and after ejaculation because the prostate contracts during orgasm to push the seminal fluid out through the penis. If he hasn't ejaculated for several days, spasms of the inflamed prostate will hurt because his prostate is full of accumulated fluid.

Diagnosing Prostatitis

You'll start with giving a urine specimen to rule out a bladder infection. Your physician will also insert a gloved finger into your rectum to examine the prostate through the rectal wall. A swollen prostate that feels warm to the touch and whimpers or screams in pain upon contact probably has some sort of infection. To know which germ is responsible, a lab must look at ejaculate fluid under a microscope, but bacteria may not be visible. Therefore, many physicians think that the presence of white blood cells in ejaculate fluid is sufficient evidence of a bacterial infection to begin antibiotics, although they don't know specifically which germ is there.

Prostate massage to obtain a purer specimen of prostatic fluid for laboratory analysis to diagnose the specific germ is a somewhat controversial procedure. Massage involves milking the prostate through the rectal wall and catching the fluid that drips out through the tip of the penis on a cotton swab. Some physicians refuse to do this, believing that prostate massage can push bacteria into the bloodstream and cause a life-threatening total-body infection called sepsis. On the other hand, some physicians believe that the only accurate way to diagnose prostatitis and prescribe the right antibiotic for the particular bacterium causing the infection is to express secretions for analysis. The initial laboratory look under the microscope may not reveal any bacteria, but by growing a culture for a few days, a laboratory technologist can identity specific bacteria causing the infection.

Massage of the prostate can hurt, especially during prostatitis, but afterward your symptoms may be less severe for a while because release of the fluid lowers pressure inside the gland. It's impossible for you to massage your own prostate to obtain that kind of relief, though, and your wife shouldn't try either. The risks of injuring the prostate or moving some of the bacteria into circulation are too great. The better solution is to start having orgasms at least once a day for a while, with or without your wife's participation. Be aware that it's possible for a couple to trade infections back and forth. Unless you both are tested and treated, you can reinfect each other with yeast, sexually transmitted diseases, *Chlamydia,* and so forth.

> *Madge and I went round and round for a while over this. She'd have a vaginal infection and go to her gynecologist to get it treated. Then a few weeks later my prostate would start hurting and I'd get treated by my urologist. It never occurred to us that we were passing germs back and forth. It was only when I saw our family doctor that someone put two and two together to figure out what was going on. We both went on a course of medicine at the same time and stopped having sex for a few nights and have been problem-free ever since.*

Treatment of Prostatitis

Once your physician diagnoses a prostate infection and rules out kidney disease, a bladder infection, or other prostate problem, treatment can proceed. Only in severe cases would hospitalization to receive antibiotics intravenously (by an IV) be necessary, or if urination becomes so difficult you are unable to void (which happens if the prostate swells so much it obstructs the urinary tube). In that case your physician will place a catheter into your bladder to drain the urine, perhaps through the front of your abdomen (a "suprapubic catheter") to avoid traumatizing your prostate by forcing a foreign object through it while it's so swollen and sore.

> *I'll never forget the evening I couldn't pass water. I'd been having a little trouble for several days, but that night as hard as I would push and try to relax, I couldn't get my bladder to cooperate. After a few hours it started to get really uncomfortable. I tried running the tap water while in the bathroom to get that urge that usually makes me feel like I have to go right now. I tried peeing in the shower.*

*Nothing worked. I finally gave up and decided to go to the ER. The
doctor greased up a tube and slid it into my bladder and drained
out more than a quart of urine. It took several minutes. I have
never felt so much better in my life! He told me to see a urologist
the next day and, sure enough, my prostate was infected again.*

Your therapy will more likely simply involve taking antibiotic
pills for two to three weeks. Be sure to take all the medicine for
the full course of treatment to avoid killing off only the weakest
germs, leaving behind the stronger, more resistant germs to flare up
again, creating an even worse infection. Also increase the amount
of fluids you drink to keep the urinary system washed out.

Increase the frequency of ejaculation to daily. There's probably
no other physical condition that plenty of sexual activity can help
so much. By keeping the amount of fluid in the prostate low, pressure doesn't build up and pain is less likely. Furthermore, the
larger volume of fluid the prostate must produce for ejaculation
rinses out the prostate. As fluids are pulled from the bloodstream
to make more prostatic fluid, antibiotics also come along into the
prostate at a better rate.

Also take a sitz bath to improve circulation to the pelvis and
soothe swollen tissues. Sit in a tub of warm water at least eight
inches deep for twenty to thirty minutes. Leave the warm water
running at a slow rate so the water temperature stays sufficiently
hot (about 105 to 110 degrees F.).

Your physician may prescribe alpha blockers (also used to treat
high blood pressure) to relax muscles inside your prostate and increase blood flow, letting antibiotics work faster. Your doctor may
also suggest an anti-inflammatory medicine such as ibuprofen
(Motrin) to reduce pain and swelling, which also improves blood
flow in your prostate. Some men have fewer problems if they
avoid foods that seem to aggravate the prostate. Try reducing
consumption of acidic foods: green, leafy vegetables, and dairy
products. Some men get relief by increasing activity and limiting
time spent sitting or driving.

One of every two or three men who have prostatitis redevelop
it with such frequency that it seems to be a chronic problem.
Sometimes the original infection has lingered. In these cases peri-
odic or long-term antibiotic treatment is an option. A physician
should also examine the prostate by ultrasound for abscesses
(pockets of infection that need draining) or prostate stones.

Don't ignore signs of prostatitis. Infection can spread into your bloodstream, causing serious problems. Unfortunately, we don't entirely know how to prevent prostatitis, except to use antibiotics long-term once a man has one infection. Even surgery to remove much of the prostate improves infection rates for only about a third of the men who have it done. The best way to prevent prostatitis is good hygiene of the penis, especially the urinary opening at the tip. Don't engage in anal intercourse without a condom or let your penis brush against your wife's anal area. Urinate after sex to wash out germs that worked their way into your penis. Avoid toilet practices that may introduce germs from the rectum into the urinary opening. Bathe daily, sudsing and rinsing the tip of the penis. If you're uncircumcised, retract your foreskin and wash well under it every day.

Nonbacterial Prostatitis

When prostatitis is due to germs other than bacteria, treatment doesn't involve antibiotics. Yeast infections respond quite well to other medications, such as a onetime large dose of fluconazole (Diflucan). Viral infections are a more difficult type to diagnose. The goal of treatment is relief from pain and urinary difficulty. Getting rid of the actual infection is left to the body's own self-defense immune mechanism, which may or may not be sufficient for the purpose. It's no wonder that many men who suffer with chronic prostatitis turn to other remedies, such as herbs or other alternatives. These other options don't generally provide the relief that their suppliers claim, though, and are poorly regulated as to potency and purity. Many have undesirable effects. A powerful placebo effect helps some men, while others cannot even tell they are taking them until side effects develop.

> *I was desperate for some relief from my prostate pain and problems. I'd heard from my friends about the ordeal of surgery and wanted to put it off as long as possible. Late one night on TV I saw an infomercial for herbal remedies, including one for the prostate. I figured that it was only money, so I ordered up a batch. The stuff had ginseng, ginger root, saw palmetto, and some other things I don't remember. I took the whole bottle according to the instructions and maybe had a little improvement. It was really hard to see any big change. I guess some guys have more luck with that stuff than I do. Among my friends, though, my experience was*

pretty typical. One thing I did notice that I didn't like was that my heart would pound sometimes or feel like it was skipping beats.

NONCANCEROUS PROSTATE ENLARGEMENT

Prostate enlargement due to disorders that aren't life-threatening occurs in about half of men more than sixty years old. By ages eighty to eighty-five, almost every man's prostate is enlarged. A significant minority of men with this problem develop some urine obstruction.

The term for noncancerous prostate enlargement is "benign prostatic hyperplasia (or hypertrophy)" (BPH). Although we don't know why BPH occurs, two primary risk factors are: (1) normal to high levels of testosterone and (2) aging. BPH rarely occurs in young men and almost never happens to men who have been castrated or have had long-term blockage of testosterone production. Many men go for years without any clue that their prostates are getting bigger and becoming boggy.

Symptoms of BPH

Urinary problems arise as the prostate gland grows, putting pressure on the urinary tube that passes through it, similar to what happens when you have to blow harder to get air through a straw while you pinch the sides. With BPH it takes more effort and time to start your urine stream.

Because the bladder has to work harder, it tires more quickly and doesn't function as effectively, leaving urine still inside the bladder after voiding. If the bladder becomes irritated, you may feel the need to urinate more often, even if there's just a small amount of urine in the bladder. Urine may dribble out less forcefully. In severe cases some men lose bladder control (called "incontinence"), requiring them to wear an absorbent pad to collect leakage.

Other symptoms include urgency (a feeling that you can't manage to hold your urine until you make it to a bathroom) and "nocturia" (having to get up at night to urinate). Nocturia disrupts your sleep by awakening you every hour or two because your bladder feels as if it's full, even though it isn't. Sleep disruptions are not only annoying, they also cause irritability and difficulty concentrating the next day.

An enlarged prostate gland is also a challenge to sexual enjoyment. Men cannot blame *erection* problems on it, though, because BPH doesn't affect circulation or nerve function. Instead, the prostate affects ejaculation. As the enlarged prostate swells to an even greater size during sexual arousal, pressure on the urinary tube can become so severe that nothing can get through— not even seminal fluid. As it passes through your sperm tract, it encounters a blockage within the prostate. Since it cannot get through, orgasmic contractions force it into the bladder, a phenomenon called "retrograde ejaculation."

Retrograde ejaculation is not dangerous; it's merely a symptom. Seminal fluid pushed into the bladder just sits there until you urinate. The next time you go to the bathroom your urine may be cloudy because it contains your ejaculation. Retrograde ejaculation renders you incapable of impregnating a woman, usually not a big concern to older men. (It is possible to extract sperm from the urine if fertility is important.) What you are more likely to wonder about is whether ejaculation is essential to good orgasms. The answer is "no." The quality of orgasms remains the same, but you won't feel seminal fluid passing through your penis. The common term for this is "dry orgasm."

> *I didn't even realize I was having dry orgasms for quite a while. We always have sex at night, so when I got up to piss later, the room was dark and I couldn't see anything different about my pee. Sarah said sex wasn't as messy as it used to be, but we just figured it was because she was drier after menopause. It wasn't until she was gone for a couple of weeks to visit her sister and I was jacking off alone that I noticed nothing was coming out. I called my doctor right away and was hugely relieved to find out it wasn't any big deal. My prostate is just getting old.*

Finding Out if You Have BPH

A physician may identify silent BPH by noting that the bladder wall is thicker than normal because the bladder muscle develops as it works harder to force out the urine. Also, urine left in the bladder after voiding is a good clue that the prostate is obstructing the urinary tube. Sometimes bladder or kidney damage indicates prostate trouble.

The easiest way to initially find BPH is for your physician to feel your prostate during a rectal examination. Sometimes BPH can occur without any appreciable growth in the overall size of the prostate, though, because the swelling takes place toward the inside of the gland against the urinary tube and doesn't show up as general enlargement.

Your physician will sort through other reasons why you may be having difficulty with urination: abnormalities in anatomy, nerve damage to your bladder, diabetes, kidney stones, an infection, or medicines you may be taking for other problems that cause urinary trouble as a side effect—particularly if you have sudden trouble starting urination. Acute urine retention can result from a wide variety of medicines, including some nonprescription drugs for colds and allergies. Decongestants can prevent the opening to the bladder from relaxing adequately to permit urine to flow. Some prescription medications such as tranquilizers, nerve-blocking agents, and others bring on acute urinary retention, especially in men who already have BPH. Sometimes urine retention comes from stress, overuse of alcohol, or even having to lie still for extended periods of time.

Your physician will also check your blood and urine to assess how well your kidneys are functioning and to rule out a urinary tract infection. These symptoms can mimic prostatitis, because an infection anywhere in the internal male reproductive or urinary systems can cause difficulty urinating.

If your family physician or internist decides you need the expertise of a urologist, expect more tests. Ultrasound, also used to diagnose prostate cancer, can measure the size of the prostate. Your physician may evaluate the force of your urine stream by asking you to urinate into a pressure-sensitive device. Low pressure indicates a reduced flow possibly related to BPH.

While primarily used for problems related to the kidneys and the tubes that drain urine *to* the bladder, an intravenous pyelogram (IVP) may be useful. An IVP lets your physician see on an X ray the path your urine takes. Dye injected into one of your veins becomes visible on X ray as the kidneys filter, concentrate, and excrete it into the bladder. The IVP lets your physician see where there might be any narrowing of urinary passageways or blockage by your prostate.

Another way to see obstructions is by cystoscopy using an instrument to look directly into your bladder. A numbing medication is first squirted into the urinary opening at the tip of your penis. The physician then inserts a tiny tube with a bright light and viewing lens on it to look for blockage.

Treating BPH

Ways to treat BPH include doing nothing, medications, surgery, and several procedures to relieve the blockage without surgery. Treatment will depend on how severely affected you are. As long as you have no symptoms and your bladder and kidneys remain undamaged, there's no need to rush into anything. Only if symptoms develop that seriously interfere with your normal life do you need treatment. This stage of waiting for the development of more advanced symptoms usually begins with your physician noticing during your regular checkup when he or she performs your rectal exam that you have an enlarged prostate.

Medications. The two primary medications for BPH are both pills requiring a prescription. The first is finasteride (Proscar), which prevents testosterone from metabolizing to a form that is particularly nasty about stimulating BPH. Once you begin Proscar, you'll probably take it for the rest of your life. You won't notice relief of symptoms right away. Several months may pass before the prostate shrinks sufficiently. Furthermore, Proscar is effective in only about a third of men who take it and is quite expensive. Another medicine is terazosin hydrochloride (Hytrin), also used to control high blood pressure. Hytrin relaxes muscles in your prostate and around the lower opening of your bladder into the urinary tube, allowing urination with less effort. Hytrin takes effect quite rapidly and is more effective. Many men take both medications for years without serious side effects.

> I don't know why I waited so long to get help with my prostate. Okay, yes, I do. I'm your basic chicken about hospitals. I didn't want surgery. So I let it go until it got really bad. I finally decided nothing could be worse than getting up every hour at night to pee, having cramps inside during sex, leaking urine, etc. My doctor put me on a prescription that really helped. It was so simple. I've been lucky that the medicine is still doing a pretty good job here two years later.

Surgery. Surgery is the best long-term treatment for eliminating BPH problems. Not many men who have surgery for BPH must have the operation repeated. Those who do were quite young when they had the first operation and have lived long enough for the prostate to regrow.

In surgery for BPH the outer capsule encasing the prostate gland remains intact, very important for avoiding nerve damage leading to erectile dysfunction. Surgery has potential for complications, though, more serious than medicinal options and other procedures, such as a recovery period that can last months. However, most men find that it completely alleviates their symptoms. There are four ways by which the surgeon can remove the offending portion of the prostate gland:

- transurethral resection of the prostate (TURP)
- transurethral incision of the prostate (TUIP)
- open surgery
- laser ablation

1. **Transurethral resection of the prostate (TURP).** Most men having prostate surgery for BPH get a TURP. Before entering the hospital you will undergo several laboratory tests and a physical examination to uncover any problems that may complicate the surgery. You will then receive a general anesthetic, letting you sleep during the hour-and-a-half-long operation. Your surgeon won't make an incision. To reach the prostate, he or she will slide a long tubular instrument through the urinary opening at the tip of your penis up to your prostate. Inside the tube is an electrical wire that delivers a tiny current to cut the tissue and stop bleeding from any small blood vessels that start leaking. There's also a bright light and an apparatus for irrigating the tube inside the instrument. Your surgeon will slowly chip away at the offending tissue, removing a sufficient portion to achieve the desired result.

2. **Transurethral incision of the prostate (TUIP).** The TUIP is similar to a TURP, except no tissue is removed. The surgeon makes small nicks in the inner prostate gland and lower bladder. This allows the tissue to fan open like an accordion, relieving obstruction and pressure. TUIP is only for men with slightly enlarged prostates and is still new enough that we don't know if it relieves BPH permanently.

3. **Open surgical removal of the prostate.** When the prostate is extremely large or when bladder repairs are necessary, the surgeon may make a small incision for direct access to the prostate. Since the prostate is not cancerous, there is no need

to remove all of the gland, though, which would risk damage that might cause erectile dysfunction.

4. **Laser ablation.** Laser ablation starts just like a TURP, except that instead of removing bits of tissue, the surgeon directs a laser beam at the prostate. A low-wattage beam destroys the tissue, which then gradually sloughs off over the next several weeks. Some surgeons prefer a higher wattage that "vaporizes" the tissue. The first method improves urine function more slowly but is less likely to damage nerves around the prostate. Laser surgery continues to undergo evaluation and has not yet reached the same level of acceptance as the TURP.

Your postoperative course.   Expect to stay in the hospital a day or two. When you first wake up after surgery you'll find a drainage tube in your bladder. Don't be alarmed if the urine draining into the storage bag looks bloody; this is normal for a few days. Your nurse will probably irrigate your bladder to prevent blood clots from clogging your catheter. Your wife may need to learn how to do some nursing procedures for you the first few days you're home, or you can arrange for a home health nurse to visit. While the drainage catheter remains in place, your bladder may spasm occasionally. Your physician can order some medication to relieve the pain, as well as antibiotics to prevent infection at the surgical site.

> *My surgery was pretty standard for that era. It has been almost twenty years since I had it done. At that time guys getting their prostates "Roto-Rootered" had to stay in the hospital for a long time. I actually enjoyed the time off, except for the bladder spasms and pain. The worst part was the embarrassment of telling people at work who wanted to know where I'd been. It was amazing, though, that once I opened up to a few of the guys, it seemed like everyone had stories to tell about their prostates.*

Most men go home wearing the catheter and come to the doctor's office later for removal. Even then, your urine may be pink a few more days. If bleeding picks up, you see clots in your urine, or have trouble urinating, notify your physician immediately.

You can help prevent excessive bleeding. Don't resume an exercise program for a few weeks. Jostling movements, straining, or sudden jerking motions may damage your healing incision site or your internal scar. Don't drive a car for a few days or return to work until your doctor gives the okay. Drink as many fluids as you can to keep the urinary system washed out frequently. Try not to become constipated, because bearing down during bowel movements can restart bleeding. Lifting heavy objects or engaging in activities that entail a lot of vibration may also irritate your prostate.

Don't expect much relief very soon. You'll probably have a strong urine stream again rather quickly, but your internal tissues will be swollen from the trauma of surgery for a while and may not function as well as you would like for a few weeks.

Sexual function after surgery for BPH. When it's time to reactivate your sex life, don't confuse stories you've heard about surgery for prostate cancer with what to expect after surgery for BPH. The most significant difference is that the surgical treatment of cancer requires removal of the entire prostate gland, presenting a greater risk for nerve damage causing permanent erectile dysfunction.

With surgery for BPH the outer capsule of the prostate gland remains untouched because only the inner portion putting pressure on the urethra needs removal. Since the nerves that promote erectile function run along the outside of the prostate, surgery for BPH has no effect on erections. This is not to say that an enlarged prostate has no sexual impact at all or that surgery to alleviate troublesome tissue has no sexual implications. After surgery for BPH the urinary tract and prostate gland are somewhat swollen and irritated, in addition to the fact that the internal scars will take a few weeks to heal.

Typically, a man won't be interested in resuming sexual activity after BPH surgery for at least a couple of weeks, which is good because the prostate needs to heal before sexual arousal makes it swell. While it's normal to feel some concern about sex, it's important not to expect sexual trouble, because this can promote "spectatoring" (see chapters 3 and 4) and erection problems. If you were able to achieve erections before surgery, you can afterward, too, within twelve weeks or so, unless psychologically hampered. Occasionally men who've lost interest in sex or doubt their remaining potential use prostate surgery as an excuse to stop sexual activity.

Every man should have his first postoperative orgasm alone. By masturbating he can take his time and notice any differences in sensations, and provide the stimulation he needs without worrying about his wife accidentally causing pain. The first orgasm after surgery is a reassuring milestone.

Surgery for BPH will not restore lost sexual function. *The exception to this* is the man whose dysfunction came out of fear of prostate pain during orgasms. As he heals and as pain gradually disappears, he may learn to stop dreading sex and relax. Otherwise, BPH surgery only relieves pressure inside the prostate. It doesn't improve or restore blood flow for erections.

I began having erection problems because my prostate started to hurt whenever I got turned on. I could really feel it swell in there. Then during orgasm sometimes it would feel like a tiny charley horse, only I couldn't massage it or stretch it out like a leg muscle to make it stop. It's surprising I kept up with sex as long as I did. I mean, who wants pain on purpose when you can avoid it? Louise gently persuaded me to try it again a few months after my operation. I still had trouble with erections, but discovered on my own that coming didn't make me hurt inside. Gradually we were able to rebuild our sex life, and I haven't had any trouble since.

One aspect of sex that *is* usually different after surgery is there will be little or no ejaculate fluid. (Many men will already be used to this, since they'd been having retrograde ejaculations before their operations.) With the removal of prostatic tissue, the gland no longer produces as much fluid as before. Also, the surgery may have cut the internal sphincter (a ring of muscle at the bottom of the bladder that normally prevents sperm from shooting upward into the bladder during orgasm). Without a functioning internal sphincter, seminal fluid is likely to flow harmlessly into the bladder rather than down through the penis, because there is lower pressure upward.

In summary, the sexual implications of a TURP should be relatively minor. Even though the prostate is important to reproduction, a TURP doesn't alter erectile function.

Nonsurgical procedures. For the man who doesn't yet want surgery, but for whom medicines aren't proving to be satisfactory, there are new options. For example, techniques used to open blocked arteries may prove effective in opening a blocked urinary tube. Studies are under way on the effectiveness of stents—tiny, springlike devices placed inside the narrowed portion of the urinary tube to push back the tissue around the blocked area. In another procedure, balloon urethroplasty, the physician inserts a catheter with a tiny deflated balloon on it through the urinary opening in the penis up to the blocked portion. The balloon then inflates, pressing open the urethra. The balloon must be removed before urination can occur, of course. This technique is not a long-term solution but is safe and can provide relief for a few months.

A technique having mixed results involves heating the prostate gland from the inside, creating a wider opening for the urine by destroying some of the prostatic tissue. A urologist does this with microwaves through a special catheter, heating targeted prostate sections to about 110 degrees F. Transurethral microwave thermotherapy (TUMT) is quite safe and doesn't usually require hospitalization. It's a relatively painless procedure and requires no anesthesia. There is little blood loss and no erectile dysfunction or loss of bladder control. However, TUMT doesn't alleviate all symptoms of BPH.

CANCER OF THE PROSTATE

According to the American Cancer Society, 58 percent of men with prostate cancer discover it while it's still confined to the prostate gland. Ninety-nine percent of these men are alive five years later. Regardless of how advanced the cancer was when discovered, the five-year survival rate for all men with prostate cancer has increased since the late 1960s from 50 percent to 87 percent.

Prostate cancer is the most frequent type affecting male Americans (except for skin cancers), responsible for more than 40 percent of all cancers in men. About forty thousand men in the United States die annually from it. The prostate is the second most frequent source of cancer-related male deaths—lung cancer being number one. How common this disease is shows up in autopsies of men more than fifty years of age: 30 percent have tiny areas of prostate cancer of which they were unaware. Overall, the lifelong risk of developing prostate cancer severe enough to cause symptoms is about 13 percent. About as many men die from it as women die from breast cancer.

Prostate cancer usually grows very slowly, often taking ten years to reach significance. On occasion, though, it can advance rapidly and requires aggressive therapy. Of men more than seventy years old who have small areas of prostate cancer, fewer than 15 percent die from it over the next ten years. Because of slow growth, it's more likely to affect older men after fifty-five, with seventy-two years being the average age of diagnosis. More than 80 percent of cases appear in men more than sixty-five years of age.

We don't know what causes prostate cancer, only some related factors. First, African American men develop it 66 percent more often than white men and die at twice the rate. If the cancer is caught early, while it's still contained within the prostate, 90 percent of these African American men are still alive five years later. Second, prostate cancer appears slightly more often in some families. If your father or your brother have or had this disease, be especially diligent in screening for it.

Men who eat high-fat diets and inadequate amounts of fruits and vegetables may be at greater risk. Prostate cancer is most common in North America and the British Isles than in other parts of the world. Inconclusive evidence suggests that occupational hazards may contribute to prostate cancer, such as work in rubber factories or with cadmium metal in battery production, electroplating, and so forth.

We do know what does *not* cause prostate cancer. Having other prostate problems, including prostate enlargement (BPH) or prostatitis, does not correlate with a higher incidence of prostate cancer. For a while another myth circulating was that vasectomies cause it. That's not true either.

Symptoms of Prostate Cancer

One of the bad things about this disease is that you probably won't have any symptoms until it has already spread beyond the prostate. Therefore it's extremely important to have regular physical examinations and screenings for it. Sometimes weight loss is the first sign of cancer. Other symptoms are similar to BPH or prostatitis because as the prostate grows with cancer, it begins to put pressure on the urethra. These include a weaker urinary flow, difficulty starting urination, having to get up frequently at night to urinate, losing bladder control, and painful ejaculation. As the cancer becomes more advanced, blood may appear in the urine or ejaculate fluid. Pain and stiffness develop in the pelvis, lower back, thighs, and hips. Surprisingly, pain of the prostate itself is not typical except possibly during orgasm, because the prostate nerves refer pain to other body parts.

Diagnosing Prostate Cancer

There's no cure for prostate cancer once it has spread, making frequent screening extremely important because chances for survival increase dramatically by catching it early.

> When I used to think about prostate cancer, I thought of Bill Bixby. Several years ago he went public with his fight against it, and for some reason he made a big impression on me. I guess I had always liked his TV shows and was floored when he died. Something just clicked inside me and made it personal. I started getting yearly exams for prostate cancer. Two years ago my doctor got back an abnormal PSA test. We had caught my cancer very early. Thanks to Bill Bixby, I expect to live to be a very old man.

The American Urological Association has set forth guidelines for prostate screening. Men in higher-risk groups should begin tests annually at forty to forty-five years of age. Those without risk factors should begin by age fifty.

Since prostate cancer eventually appears in most men as they get closer to their elderly years but they usually die from something else, there comes a point at which routine screening may no longer be worthwhile. The difficulty is knowing at what age this is. Generally speaking, a healthy seventy-year-old with responsibilities and an active lifestyle would certainly want to continue annual prostate screening, whereas another seventy-year-old in poor health who probably won't live another five to ten years could relax in regard to the possibility of prostate cancer seriously affecting him.

If cancer is suspected, your physician will examine your urine for signs of blood or infection and may require an IVP or cystoscopy (see explanations of these procedures in "Finding Out if You Have BPH" earlier in this chapter) to rule out other problems in the urinary system. To accurately identify cancer, though, there are four steps to diagnosis: a rectal examination, the prostate specific antigen test (PSA), a transrectal ultrasound, and a biopsy.

Rectal examination.   The traditional way to detect prostate cancer has been for your physician to feel your prostate through the rectal wall. Normally the prostate feels slightly spongy, like the pads of your fingertips. The cancer tumor feels like a hard nodule, more like your knuckle feels. Other clues are irregularity in shape, lumpiness, or dimpling. Unfortunately, by the time tumors in the prostate become large enough to feel, more than half the cases of prostate cancer have already spread to lymph nodes or bones.

Prostate specific antigen (PSA).   The PSA is a simple blood test that dramatically improves the discovery rate of prostate cancer. PSA is a substance made only by prostate gland cells. As the cancer grows and may spread into bones, lymph nodes, and other body parts, PSA in the bloodstream increases. The higher the PSA, the more advanced the cancer is. Since no other type of cancer makes PSA, the test is specific for this particular disease. The test can reveal as many as 80 percent of cases of prostate cancer, reducing deaths significantly by catching the disease early enough for treatment to still work.

However, the PSA test is not perfect. About a third of men who have abnormally high PSA amounts don't have cancer. Factors that cause the PSA level to rise include prostate infection, BPH (noncancerous enlargement), a recent bladder infection, or even a prostate evaluation. Therefore your physician should have your blood drawn before the rectal exam. PSA also increases as a man ages because his prostate grows.

Sexual activity, too, raises the PSA because more PSA seeps into circulation when the prostate spasms during orgasm. Therefore, abstain from sex for at least two days before your PSA test to avoid a falsely high level that would require you to undergo further tests.

Generally speaking, a normal PSA should be below 4.0 nanograms per milliliter (4.0 ng/ml) of blood. It should be below 2.5 for men in their forties, and below 6.5 for men in their seventies. When cancer is extensive, the PSA can climb as high as 1,000 ng/ml. Urologists can also use the PSA to calculate the odds that the cancer has spread beyond the prostate. If the PSA ranges between 10 and 20 ng/ml, there is approximately a 25 percent likelihood that the cancer remains confined to the prostate. If more than 20 ng/ml, they are quite confident it has spread.

Once cancer is diagnosed, PSA tests help monitor success of treatment. After surgical removal of the prostate, the PSA should drop to almost zero. With radiation treatment it will probably take several months, or even a couple of years, for the PSA level to return to normal. A rising PSA is a clue the cancer is starting to regrow. Therefore, even men who've apparently been treated successfully for prostate cancer need to continue screening for recurrence.

Transrectal ultrasound and prostate biopsy. The next step and the only certain way to determine if you have prostate cancer is to confirm it by examining prostate cells under a microscope. To get these cells, your physician must do a biopsy—that is, remove a tiny piece of tissue from the prostate, using a hollow needle. A biopsy usually takes fewer than thirty minutes and is quite painless.

To properly identify where to get cell specimens, your physician will first examine your prostate using an ultrasound machine by sliding into your rectum a small probe that sends out sound waves humans cannot hear. As the sound waves bounce off tissues, a computer transfers the information into a picture called a sonogram. Your physician uses the picture to guide the biopsy needle to the right place, taking at least six specimens, one from each of the primary areas of the prostate, plus cells from any known tumors.

This procedure has no side effects other than possibly some slight rectal discomfort, or tiny amounts of blood in your urine or bowel movements for a few days. Transrectal ultrasound and biopsy do not require hospitalization or anesthesia. Preparations include stopping any medication for a few days that would make you more prone to bleeding during the procedure, such as aspirin or warfarin (Coumadin). The morning of your test you'll also give yourself a small enema to clear the rectum (the Fleet brand works well). After the test you'll probably take antibiotics as a precaution against infection.

> *I know it sounds weird now, but at the time I was more worried about having something up my butt than I was about cancer. I just couldn't imagine anything more humiliating. Everyone at the hospital was so professional, though. They really treated me with respect and protected my modesty. We joked about stuff, I was made as comfortable as possible, and everyone there acted like they did this every day (which they do) and it was no different than doing an eye exam. It was over quite fast and I was really glad I hadn't backed out.*

If the biopsy reveals you do indeed have prostate cancer, you'll receive a Gleason's score, indicating how severe it is. Cancer cells are rated from 1 to 5 based on how they look, with the most aggressive types of cancer cells getting a score of 5. A pathologist will also score the second most common type of cancer cells you have and add it to the first score, yielding a final Gleason score of as much as 10 if your cancer is of the most serious type. Most men have a score of 5 to 6. About a third of men with prostate cancer have a score of 7 to 10.

The next step is to determine if the cancer has spread (metastasized) by undergoing bone-scan or lymph node biopsies. Two different systems indicate how far prostate cancer has advanced: the TNM (tumor-nodes-metastasis) and the Whitmore. The TNM method is rather complicated, whereas in Whitmore staging, an A or a B means the cancer is still confined within the prostate, a C means it has spread to nearby areas, and a D means it's now in more distant body parts.

Treatment Options

For men still healthy in most other respects and with a life expectancy of at least ten more years, surgery is the best choice. Older men might choose to have radiation therapy instead. There is no statistical evidence to show that either method is better for prolonging life. Some physicians even recommend just waiting to see how rapidly the cancer advances. Since prostate cancer usually grows quite slowly, waiting is not as risky as with other types of cancer. You can certainly take at least a few weeks to look into your choices and think about them carefully. Consider the financial expense, risk to your general health and sexual function, side effects, emotional trauma, and how much each therapy will force you to change your lifestyle.

One consideration must be, of course, whether the cancer is confined to the prostate or has spread. For cancer caught early, surgery and radiation therapy are acceptable. However, if the cancer has metastasized, these are still possible *partial* treatments, but other choices include hormone therapy, chemotherapy, and perhaps even alternative medicines. While none of these last options can cure cancer, they may slow its growth and provide some relief from unpleasant symptoms.

Once your family physician or urologist has diagnosed cancer, it may be necessary to also bring additional specialists on board your health care team. While the urologist can do your surgery and monitor any hormone therapy, you might also need the services of an oncologist, a physician who specializes in the treatment of cancer, to direct radiation treatments or chemotherapy. Let's review each treatment option and the sexual implications.

1. **Watchful waiting.** Doing nothing might be especially attractive to you if you know your cancer is in its early stages and is a slow-growing type, which a low Gleason score would tell you. An elderly man whose health is seriously impaired or who probably won't live more than ten more years would be wise to think twice about aggressively treating something that probably won't kill him.

   With watchful waiting it is important not to forget the *watchful* part, meaning that PSA tests and rectal exams are necessary at least every three months to catch any clues that the cancer may be growing or spreading. If signs of advancing cancer appear, then other treatment options are still available. In countries where the government operates a nationalized health service in which the population gets "free" health care paid by taxes, watchful waiting is often the only choice offered.

2. **Radical prostatectomy**

   Surgical choices. When cancer is still confined to the prostate gland, the usual treatment is a radical prostatectomy. For this, the surgeon must remove the entire gland to be sure to get all the cancer. Therefore, the types of operations used for noncancerous enlargement of the prostate (BPH) aren't useful because they remove only the inner portion of the gland.

   A radical prostatectomy requires an incision to visualize the entire organ and remove it completely. The prostate encircles the urethra, so a small portion of the urinary tube has to come out, too, which the surgeon reconnects to the bladder. Since cancer often spreads next into lymph nodes, those may be excised, too. The procedure takes two to four hours, plus preoperative preparation time and recovery from general anesthesia.

   The incision can be made in two possible places. The easiest and traditional route is through the perineum, the area behind the scrotum in front of the anus. This "perineal prostatectomy" is better for the surgeon because the prostate is closer to the surface there, and it's easier to reattach the urethra. Recovery is usually quicker. There are two problems, though. One is that sometimes an abdominal incision is still necessary to get all the lymph nodes. Second, and even more distressing, is that the perineal route is more likely to cut nerves responsible for stimulating erections. Most men having this procedure lose erectile function permanently.

> *When my dad had his prostate taken out thirty years ago, he didn't say anything about what he sacrificed to fight the cancer. When I discovered prostate cancer last year, though, he finally opened up to me about how he and Mom lost an important part of their relationship because his surgery left him impotent. He had heard about the new techniques and wanted to make sure I had, too. He isn't bitter anymore, but just said that no man should have to make those kinds of choices (to live without sex or to die).*

The newer route, a "retropubic prostatectomy," is better for sexual reasons. The surgeon makes the incision in the front of the lower abdomen and gets to the prostate by going over the pubic bone and below the bladder. Not only does the retropubic route make lymph node removal easier, it also avoids nerves in the perineum. In addition to using this route, though, the surgeon must also use a technique called "nerve sparing" to preserve as much sexual function as possible (see the upcoming section on sexual implications and adjustment after a prostatectomy).

Recovering from a radical prostatectomy. When you wake up from surgery you will have a catheter to drain urine from your bladder. You can probably go home in two or three days. The urinary catheter will stay in place several days longer so the internal surgical site can heal, particularly the area where your urinary tube was reattached to your bladder.

Within a month you'll probably be back to most of your usual activities, although you should start gradually. Full strength returns within three or four months. This is not to say that everything about your urinary system will function fully that soon. Urinary leakage is inevitable for at least several weeks. Loss of bladder control (incontinence) can continue for a minority of men for as long as a year, depending on how extensively the surgery traumatized the bladder. Even after a year some men still have stress incontinence, unintentional urine loss when pressure increases in the abdomen from coughing, lifting heavy objects, sneezing, or even laughing. Fortunately, permanent severe incontinence is rare.

Sexual implications and adjustment after a prostatectomy. Even if your surgery is by the retropubic route, there can be sexual nerve damage. Ask for "nerve sparing" surgery. Investigate the surgeon's success rate for protecting erectile function. Be aware, too, though, that nerve-sparing surgery is usually available only to men whose cancer tumors are small and well confined.

A nerve-sparing prostatectomy protects the bundles of nerves and blood vessels running along the outside of the prostate that are important for penile erection ability. The surgeon must carefully loosen the covering around the prostate, and remove the prostate while leaving the covering intact. Since nerves important to sexual function are difficult to isolate, research is under way to develop technology that will electrically stimulate them during the operation so surgeons can identify which ones to avoid.

In a nerve-sparing prostatectomy, the nerves at greatest risk are those supplying the corpora cavernosa (the two primary spongy bodies in the penis that fill with blood and create an erection). However, even if your prostatectomy renders you permanently incapable of an erection, all is not lost. You can get a penile implant to produce erections for intercourse or explore other options (see chapter 4). Furthermore, other nerves that transmit sensations to and from your penis and that orgasm may remain functional. You should still be able to feel penile stimulation and have orgasms.

Some men become so disheartened at not being able to have erections anymore that they automatically assume they're also incapable of orgasms. Others have heard stories from men who had prostatectomies many years ago who totally lost all erectile function, and expect the same thing will happen to them. Some take the surgeon's warning about the possibility of losing erections as fact, and feel there's no use trying. It's impossible to know how many haven't even attempted to resume sex because of this faulty assumption.

While it may seem odd to continue stimulation of a flaccid penis, that's exactly what it takes to build sexual arousal to orgasm, even though the penis never hardens or lengthens. (Of course, ejaculation will not accompany the orgasm since the prostate gland is gone. Even if you retain erectile function after a prostatectomy, you will still have "dry orgasms.") Give yourself permission to maximize the remaining sexual abilities you do have. The pleasurable sensations of orgasms remain strong. Give yourself a sufficient amount of time to see if erectile function returns on its own.

> *Violet and I had many problems, but sex wasn't one of them. We were determined that no matter what happened because of my prostate surgery, we were going to find a way to keep on having a good sex life. When my operation left me impotent, I just couldn't accept it—and neither could Violet. We started reading and asking everyone we could find who was willing to talk about what to do. We experimented with what we could still manage. Sometimes she could stuff my limp penis inside of her, but we couldn't really move much without it falling out. I found that sexual stimulation still felt good and wondered whether I could have an orgasm if we could just get the erection going. We tried the vacuum pump and the rubber band thing but thought there had to be something better. After thinking about it for several months and consulting a sex therapist, we decided to go ahead with the implant and have never regretted it. Now Vi plays with me a little, I pump up, and we start intercourse. Not only is she thrilled, but I've had pretty good success at having orgasms during intercourse.*

If, on the other hand, you and your wife decide that you're willing to adjust your sexual habits and live without erections, you can do that, too. Explore new ways of interacting sexually. You can have very positive results in ways you never thought possible. Your sexual repertoire will expand, giving your sex life a kick by introducing new techniques that are quite revitalizing. For example, your wife will discover that oral sex takes less effort for her. The flaccid penis fits into her mouth more easily, and she will be able to continue stimulation longer. She can also massage your penis by hand, using a lubricant.

If you both want to continue intravaginal sexual stimulation, particularly in conjunction with clitoral stimulation, use a dildo (an artificial penis) or slip one or two fingers into her vagina to provide the friction and pressure that is pleasurable to her. Don't simply abandon sex. You need to stay sexually active for better psychological health and a happier marital relationship. Also, your wife physically needs intravaginal massage by some method to keep her vagina free from adhesions.

> *Leonard's prostate cancer was discovered very early, so we're quite confident he is cured. His surgery did leave him impotent, though. We had been enjoying an active sex life until then, even though we're now in our sixties. Sex had been such an important part of our relationship that we began experimenting with new ways to keep it going. I started giving Leo blow jobs with pretty spectacular success, but I missed having something in my vagina. He wasn't revved up about getting a penis implant, though. After some serious discussion he suggested that we "go modern" and try some sex toys. I was game, but concerned that he might resent using a fake penis. I was very surprised that his reaction was just the opposite. He got a voyeuristic charge out of it. He said that in some ways it was better than before, because it was less exhausting for him than intercourse, and he had a better view. We always were good at making life's lemons into lemonade.*

One of the most important factors determining how much sexual function you'll retain after a prostatectomy, other than whether surgery cut important nerves, is how well you functioned sexually before surgery. Don't expect a prostatectomy to improve circulation or to strengthen the hardness of erections. It won't.

Furthermore, even if you had nerve-sparing surgery, those nerves will still be traumatized for several weeks, causing some temporary erectile difficulty. Abstain from sexual activity for three to four weeks anyway, because your incision may reopen, or bleeding may begin around the base of the bladder. Once you do resume sex, try not to expect even average performance for a while. Don't be discouraged, and don't try harder to have an erection, since you may create a psychological dysfunction (see chapter 4) that will mask the eventual recovery of your nerves. Relax and let yourself recover from surgery.

The psychological link to erectile dysfunction explains why some men who've had nerve-sparing surgery but experience erectile dysfunction respond amazingly well later to treatments such as Viagra. Viagra doesn't reconnect cut nerves; it only improves blood flow into the penis. However, taking Viagra gives some men the psychological strength needed to overcome a dysfunction, because they place confidence in the Viagra pill rather than in their own efforts. This is not a derogatory observation. The placebo effect *is* very valuable, and anything that safely helps restore sexual ability is worthwhile. These men may find eventually that they need Viagra less often as sexual confidence returns.

There's another explanation why Viagra works for some men who blamed their lost erections on their prostatectomies, even with nerve-sparing surgery. At first, erectile function may have been lost because of discouragement during recovery, when the nerves saved were still not working well because of surgical trauma to the tissues. Later, although the nerves were working well, circulatory problems began blocking arteries to the penis. Since the nerves were fine, all these men needed was some Viagra to open the blood vessels to restore erections.

3. **Cryotherapy.** Cryotherapy (or cryosurgery) uses liquid nitrogen or carbon dioxide, substances so extremely cold they instantly freeze tissue on contact. For prostate cancer a surgeon might use cryotherapy to freeze the diseased prostate tissue. To reach the prostate, the surgeon slides a probe into the perineum behind the scrotum and injects the freezing chemical through a hollow tube. Instead of removing the prostate, over several weeks the body gradually absorbs the destroyed tissue.

    Cryotherapy is a new procedure still under evaluation. It's certainly not valuable if cancer has already spread, but may be a good option when health problems negate surgery. It can be difficult to control how far the freezing effect reaches, so there has been a high incidence of erectile dysfunction and urinary incontinence after cryotherapy, usually for not more than a few weeks.

4. **Radiation therapy.** Radiation therapy involves beaming high-
   energy radioactive rays toward the body parts where cancer is.
   It's effective because cancer cells grow faster and absorb
   more radiation than normal cells do. Therefore, they're more
   likely to die from radiation than normal cells are.

   Radiation is potentially useful at any stage of prostate cancer. When cancer is still early, radiation can be as effective as
   surgery, at least for ten years after treatment. Beyond that
   time, though, cure rates aren't as good. Men who undergo
   prostatectomy and have a recurrence of the cancer find that it
   usually appears within the first four years or so after surgery.
   With radiation, though, recurrence can take place over many
   more years, since the prostate wasn't removed and radiation
   may not have destroyed all cancer cells.

   With radiation there are no surgical risks, such as bleeding
   or infection. Hospitalization is much shorter (if necessary at
   all) and recovery is faster. Since the prostate and the lymph
   nodes stay intact, there is less certainty about the progress of
   the disease, though. Generally your physician will monitor
   your PSA frequently to determine how effective therapy is
   and to catch any sign that the cancer might be recurring.

   Radiation can also help after a prostatectomy as a precaution in destroying cancer cells that may have spread to lymph
   nodes. Furthermore, when prostate cancer has spread to
   other body parts, radiation can slow growth of tumors and
   help relieve pain, particularly in the bones.

   How radiation therapy is given.   Radiation can be administered by directing a beam from an external source or by using
   tiny implants called "seeds" placed directly inside the prostate.
   You can receive external radiation without hospitalization, but
   you'll need to come for treatments at least five days a week
   for up to six weeks. This way the radiation dose doesn't have
   to be so high each day, rather than zapping the cancer for a
   shorter time with more energy, causing more severe side effects. With external-beam radiation you won't need anesthesia
   and won't feel much if anything during treatment.

   Expect side effects to appear within a few days. Your skin
   around the beam's targeted area may become dry, inflamed,
   and tender. Many people lose some or all of their pubic hair

temporarily. The bladder and the rectum often become sore and hypersensitive from radiation, as shown by blood in the urine or bowel movements, diarrhea, flatulence (rectal gas), painful and frequent urination, or a burning sensation in the rectum. Most people don't have these problems, but they are severe for a few. Virtually everyone experiences considerable fatigue. Reduce your workload and get more rest while staying as involved in normal activities as you can.

The other type of radiation therapy involves placing pellets, also called interstitial implants (or "seeds"), inside the prostate. Brachytherapy is a variation, delivering radiation to the prostate with radioactive needles. To position the implants properly, your physician will first do an ultrasound (sonogram) of your prostate to determine where your tumor is. A computer-generated map guides placement of about forty to a hundred seeds through a hollow tube inserted behind your scrotum through your perineum. The seeds contain radioactive iridium, iodine, or palladium. After the procedure, which usually lasts less than an hour, you can go home that same day as soon as you recover from the general anesthetic.

Your physician will probably leave the radiation seeds in your body permanently. The amount of radiation they produce decreases gradually, but even during their most potent period they aren't dangerous to others except possibly for extended, continuous periods. Assure your wife that the implants won't dislodge and be ejaculated. The radiation won't affect her. As a precaution, it's best not to let your pelvis remain in *prolonged* close contact with someone else for the first couple of months, though. You certainly can hold your grandchildren on your lap, but shouldn't let them fall asleep and stay there for several hours.

The side effects of internal implants are the same as for external radiation but are sometimes more severe because of continual radiation. Of particular note is the higher incidence of rectal pain. However, internal implants require only one hospital visit and are more convenient. Both methods have about the same cure rates.

Sexual implications of radiation therapy.   Men who opt for radiation implants can resume sexual activity within a few days. At first there may be a small amount of blood in the ejaculate fluid, a normal side effect from insertion of the implants into the prostate. Bleeding should stop in a few days. Some men have ejaculation pain that subsides with time. Again, radiation seeds don't dislodge and cannot be ejaculated.

Erection problems occur surprisingly often, considering there is no surgical trauma to the nerves. Up to half of men getting radiation have erectile dysfunction at least for a while. This may be due to severe fatigue, but more likely is due to irritation of nerves along the prostate that stimulate erection.

Sperm production can drop, and some sperm take on abnormal shapes. The cells that form sperm within the testes operate at a high metabolic rate and are more likely to absorb radiation than other body cells are. Sometimes testosterone production drops, too, explaining temporary loss of sex drive and decreased erections. Generally, once radiation therapy stops or the implants lose their potency, sperm and testosterone production returns to normal levels. Sperm forms may continue to be abnormal, however. If you plan to father more children, consider banking your sperm for later use before undergoing radiation.

5. **Hormone therapy.** Because testosterone promotes prostate cancer growth, the goal of hormone therapy is to prevent cancer cells and the prostate from receiving the male hormones that stimulate them. Without testosterone, the cancer may even shrink in size for at least a couple of years. Usually symptoms subside and the man feels better. Eventually, though, the cancer becomes active again.

Hormone therapy is a palliation for prostate cancer, not a cure. It's generally reserved for cases when cancer has already metastasized and other treatments have failed. No therapy can cure prostate cancer after hormone treatments no longer help. Sometimes men choose this method of treatment when the discovery of cancer comes so late that surgery or radiation holds little hope. There are four primary ways by which your physician can stop the effect of testosterone on your cancer:

- prevent the testes from making testosterone
- administer antiandrogen medicines
- use the female hormone estrogen to block testosterone
- remove the source of testosterone

First, luteinizing hormone-releasing hormone (LHRH) ago-nists, such as Lupron and Zolodex, stop testosterone production. LHRH agonists are injected every one to three months. They are quite expensive but have few side effects, other than what you would expect to happen when anything reduces testosterone. A common problem is loss of sex drive. They sometimes cause a "tumor flare," when cancer growth temporarily increases and symptoms get worse for a while. Taking an antiandrogen for several months can reduce the severity of this reaction.

Second, antiandrogen pills taken every day block the action of small amounts of testosterone remaining. These include flu-tamide (Eulexin) and bicalutamide (Casodex). Antiandrogens do little to lengthen survival, though. Side effects include nau-sea, breast enlargement, and decreased libido.

Third, the female hormone estrogen (usually taken as di-ethylstilbestrol [DES]) overrides testosterone. Estrogen is in-expensive but does increase risk of heart attacks and blood clots, especially in the legs. Estrogen also feminizes the male body, as shown by breast tenderness and enlargement.

Fourth, the most radical step is surgical removal of the testes, the primary producers of testosterone. This surgery (orchiectomy) is the same thing as castration. Although it's an extreme measure to take, by this point the man's life is in se-rious jeopardy. Having an orchiectomy can increase his sur-vival by several months. Orchiectomy can be a "last resort" effort or a way of skipping the above hormone therapies.

With each method of hormone therapy, some men experi-ence hot flashes, not unlike those women have during meno-pause. These aren't dangerous, but can be uncomfortable and inconvenient.

The sexual implications of hormone therapy are by far more serious. The first symptom is loss of sex drive. Some-times libido has already diminished due to the effects of ad-vanced cancer, fatigue, and pain. As testosterone production stops, erectile ability gradually disappears, too. Sexual plea-sure does remain an anatomic possibility. At this stage what the husband sometimes needs more than orgasms, though, is affection, comfort, intimacy, and companionship. He can still help his wife meet her sexual needs by encouraging her to stay as sexually active as she can. They can do this together through clitoral stimulation and use of a dildo.

By the time David decided to have his testicles taken out, we were desperate. I just couldn't let him go yet. He saw that step as the last straw in a long series of disheartening and painful tries and figured "Why not?" Sure, he lost his sex drive, but we learned so much together in those last few months about how far true love can go. I know he did it for me. Losing his male hormones didn't destroy his masculinity anyway. He was still the same old Dave. He continued to show such love and courage and strength. And he was sexy until the end, even without being as sexual.

6. **Chemotherapy.** Chemotherapy isn't effective against prostate cancer, particularly once it has spread. Some physicians try Adriamycin or Cisplatinum anyway because occasionally chemotherapy helps reduce symptoms, especially bone pain. See chapter 8 for more information about chemotherapy.

Be Prepared

Since there's no way to prevent prostate cancer, the best plan is to catch it as early as possible. For more information call the Prostate Cancer Support Network at 1-800-248-7866, the Prostate Health Council at 1-800-242-2383, or the American Cancer Society at 1-800-227-2345.

8

THE SEXUAL CHALLENGES OF CANCER

The meaning of cancer has changed considerably. Fifty years ago, when family members heard that Dad had cancer, their first question was, "How long does he have to live?" The diagnosis of cancer was synonymous with a death sentence because we had little hope for stopping it. With the wonderful advances in early cancer detection, the increasing sophistication of the field of oncology as a specialty, and newly emerging cancer drugs, the question today is typically, "What can Dad do to continue living as normal a life as possible?" Since people with cancer can now be more optimistic, the focus is turning to improving the quality of survival. One of the key aspects of a life worth living is sexual happiness.

SEXUAL CONCERNS REGARDING CANCER

Factors Affecting Sexual Adjustment

Several influences predict how well a person will cope with cancer and adjust sexually: age and stage of life; gender; the personal value placed on the affected body parts; the sexual success of the marriage before the diagnosis of cancer; the attitudes of other people; and the availability of role models.

Age and stage of life.   The person who has already lived long enough to have encountered other challenges to health or body image is more likely to have a smoother ride through the crisis of cancer. If we've already met most of our life goals, we're less likely to grieve a potentially fatal diagnosis. The more often we have learned how to change and grow and adapt, the better we get at it.

Gender.   Men and women tend to react to cancer differently, particularly because of how illness changes roles and affects our perceptions of our bodies. Whenever our bodies fail and prevent us from fulfilling our normal male or female roles, or when they alter our gender-based values, the result can seriously hamper sexual feelings. In some ways women cope with cancer better than men do because sickness seems to be more acceptable for women than for men. Health limitations can be a bigger shock to a man's ego. Some men feel demasculinized by illness. However, women are usually more psychologically vulnerable to illnesses that alter physical appearance, as cancer and its treatments sometimes do.

The personal value placed on the affected body parts.   We all have favorite physical features that we like about ourselves. Some people think their smile is their best asset. For others it's their eyes, hair, muscles, waistline, breasts, buttocks, penis, or other part. If that feature changes significantly, we may lose our feelings of attractiveness.

> *I'd always thought my best physical quality was my hair. It was long and thick and shiny. I was one of those fortunate people who never had a "bad hair day." I always got compliments about it. My husband loved for me to wear it down during lovemaking so he could run his hands through it and feel it brush against his skin as I moved. Well, one of my mother's favorite sayings was "Pride goeth before a fall," so I guess I was overdue for a little humbling. When I got cancer and had to start chemotherapy, my biggest anxiety was about my hair falling out, so I bought the best wig I could afford ahead of time. It wasn't until the night when my hair*

started to fall out in clumps, though, that the true injustice of it all hit me. I cried for a long time. Thank God, my husband was able to convince me that he loves me for more than my hair. I had never really understood how much until we went through that together.

A change in how we perceive our physical attractiveness can occur even when the shift is temporary. We merely have to suffer an alteration in our concept of that body part or a threat to its normal function, leading to feelings of embarrassment or self-consciousness. As our inner worth faces serious challenges, we believe that we're becoming less desirable to our mates. Some people withdraw from physical contact with their spouses and even avoid social events.

Since each person's self-image is unique, acceptance of change is difficult to predict. One man who has neck surgery for cancer may feel more humiliated about his scars than another man might. Some women value their breasts as their key feminine feature, while others tolerate them as nuisance appendages.

Cancer can become more than an illness to conquer. For some people it's also a source of shame and disgust. They almost feel as if they're living with a parasite or have an alien growing inside their bodies. The cancer doesn't feel like it is truly part of them. They are so mortified that they can't believe anyone else would want to be near them. This type of body image disturbance can be especially challenging. One way to overcome it is to learn what cancer really is: a change in normal cells causing them to grow too rapidly and function destructively—not an infestation or a contamination. Counseling may also help them to accept their bodies, even with its traitorous flaws, and to use positive mental imagery to reestablish feelings of self-worth.

For several weeks after I heard I had cancer I had a lot of trouble seeing it as part of me. It felt like someone was trespassing on my most private property: my body. Not just trespassing, invading me. I felt sickened at the thought—dirty, repulsed, ashamed, horrified, deformed. What was this thing growing inside of me? How could anyone want to be with me, let alone love me? What saved me was the very wise requirement my cancer center had for support group counseling. One of our exercises was to visualize the cancer as something that was part of us that we could control. We practiced loving ourselves—our whole selves. We also created im-

*ages in our minds of our bodies overcoming the cancer. I strongly
believe in the power of mental healing as part of physical healing.*

The amount of adjustment necessary also relates to how extensively the affected body part has changed. For example, upon learning they have breast cancer, most women hope for a simple "lumpectomy" over a total mastectomy (removal of the breast), because it leaves most of the breast intact, as well as more of their feelings of feminine wholeness.

The sexual success of the marriage before the diagnosis of cancer. A crisis pulls a husband and wife together and strengthens the marriage. They run to each other and cling tightly for comfort and support as they ride through the rough times. Sex becomes even more precious—a reaction much more likely when the marital relationship was strong before the crisis. Unfortunately, couples who had preexisting marital problems may find that sexual difficulties worsen after the discovery of cancer. The stress of the initial shock, changes in perceptions of each other, alterations to daily routines, financial strains, and so forth place greater tension on the relationship. While we'd like to think that the marriage vows in which we commit to stay together "in sickness and in health" would cover this contingency, the truth is that many marriages need outside assistance to endure.

The attitudes of other people.   We are all susceptible to the attitudes of people around us. Our spouses, relatives, friends, coworkers, and the people in the health care system who care for us can make all the difference in whether we continue to feel sexual and attractive. While allowing us to grieve about our condition, they must also convey a positive attitude, a sense of hope, an expectation that there is still a future worth living, and a clear message that we continue to be valued and desirable.

The most important people in this process are our spouses. They must be involved in every step of treatment and recovery as a key part of the team. Their ability to express positive feelings is important to our self-esteem and to help us keep feeling as normal as possible. For example, they mustn't let us use cancer as an excuse for closing down our sexual relationship. This may be difficult, since they also have issues through which to work. They, too, must adjust sexually and may have misconceptions about cancer.

The availability of role models. Some people with cancer never knew anyone else before who had faced the same problem—or if they did, they didn't have access to the details of their private struggles. An effective way to keep people with cancer hopeful and encouraged is for them to meet others who have coped with the same diagnosis. Their successes can be used as patterns for new victories. Their stories tell us that our feelings aren't unusual. Their tidbits of advice make our challenges easier to endure. These mentors can be found through local cancer support groups, national cancer hot lines, health care providers, and the Internet in chat rooms where other people struggle with the same problems. Your husband or wife may also benefit from discussions with other spouses about feelings and for suggestions on how to cope.

> *Perry had a big impact on me. When my wife mentioned that the hospital had someone who could come see me if I wanted to talk about how to contend with my new colostomy, I didn't really want to talk to anyone. I'd always managed with other stuff that had come up before in life and didn't want any help this time either. The night before I went home he just showed up, though. He was incredible. He told me stuff about his most embarrassing moments and all he'd learned. He even showed me his colostomy. He got me to talking about things I'd never told anyone. I'll never forget what he did for me. He helped me to feel normal again and really boosted my confidence that night.*

Sexual Worries That Often Go Unexpressed

Is it wrong to still want sex? Some people are surprised to discover that they still want sex in the midst of the upheaval of cancer. It seems strange to them that during a crisis, particularly a life-threatening one, they would still be thinking about sex. They have the impression that sex somehow seems inappropriate under the circumstances. The desire for sex is very understandable, though, because sexuality provides comfort, affirms our desirability to someone else, deepens interpersonal intimacy, conveys support, helps us feel connected during illness, and just plain feels good. Nothing about cancer erases those desires and joys. It's absolutely normal to still want sex while fighting cancer.

Will sex harm me? Another concern that worries some people considerably but that they think sounds too silly to express is whether sexual activity when one has cancer can do physical damage. One of the purposes of this chapter is to answer those concerns. Generally speaking, sex is not dangerous and actually improves psychological and physical health. We will later look at the few temporary exceptions to this related to special circumstances.

How will my spouse react to my having cancer? To answer this we must evaluate the strength of the marriage, the quality of information your spouse receives about your illness, his or her coping skills, and whether your spouse chooses to be supportive and positive. Realistically, it would be unreasonable to expect your mate to be totally optimistic. He or she will have fears of losing you and will have to make many personal adjustments by taking over some of your duties, redefining your relationship, and altering his or her own sexual patterns. Your husband or wife will also have many of the same concerns you do, such as whether sexual activity can hurt you and whether sexual feelings are inappropriate. It can seem selfish to the healthy spouse to still want sex when the partner is going through serious illness. Sexual needs and feelings are normal, though. They show us that cancer and crisis cannot destroy the essence of what still makes life worthwhile.

Can I give cancer to my spouse? Another concern for some is whether the disease is contagious. Be assured that cancer cannot pass from one person to another and is certainly not a sexually transmitted disease. It is just as likely that you would catch cancer from your spouse as it would be to catch hearing loss, a broken arm, or arthritis. It simply doesn't happen.

Why is my spouse so irritable? The emotions of the spouse of a person with cancer bounce back and forth between compassion and irritation. A wife may feel great concern one minute about her husband's well-being, then the next minute be angry because he doesn't seem to be trying anymore. Sometimes spouses can't help resenting how cancer has changed their lives, too, and then feel guilty about the resentment. In the meantime, they keenly feel that it's their responsibility to keep the person with cancer hopeful. It becomes more and more difficult for both partners to tolerate each other's periods of withdrawal or depression. They feel powerless to pull each other out of dark moods. Cancer almost feels like another person has joined the relationship and is doing everything it can to destroy equilibrium.

Sometimes people with cancer use the disease as an excuse to stop doing activities they could still manage. Some even take on an invalid or helpless mentality, adding to the strain on the well spouse. Along with this attitude of "I'm sick, so don't expect me to do anything" comes a decline in sexual interest and effort. This may be a symptom of depression. Keeping up a positive attitude and trying to push the affected spouse back into action get tiring. It's easy to cross the line into destructive nagging, which then leads to feelings of guilt and discouragement. These couples often need professional help to stop the downward spiral.

I'd have given Connie a kick in the pants if it would have helped. I've never felt so helpless in my life. She had usually been a pretty positive person, with lots of hobbies and activities. But about six months into her fight with cancer, she started to let herself go. She just didn't try anymore. The doctor said she was doing quite well physically, so I couldn't understand why she was acting so blah. She wouldn't even do the easy things that took no effort. Needless to say, our sex life was extinct. The more I pushed her, the more she resisted, and the angrier and guiltier I felt. It wasn't until her sister came to visit for a few days that the lightbulb went on. She told me that Connie was depressed and that if I didn't get her some help fast, Connie was going to go suicidal on me. Between the two of us, we got her in to see a psychiatrist. He got her on some medicine for the depression. She also joined a support group for people with cancer. Even though we haven't beaten the cancer yet, our sex life is back to normal, and Connie is doing a lot better psychologically.

Will my spouse's sexual attraction to me change if he or she becomes my caregiver?   Another common problem ensues if the healthy spouse has to function as caregiver. This role requires a unique attitude melding compassion and love with the tasks of cleaning, feeding, and assisting. It's difficult to be both a caregiver and a sexual partner for several reasons. First, performing physical caretaking tasks creates a parenting-type persona that conflicts with the sexual lover role. Usually the people in life who bathe and dress us are those with whom we don't have a sexual relationship. Our dependency on them hinders a sense of equality. We feel like passive participants or subordinates in the relationship rather than peers.

Another reason it's difficult to be a caregiver and a sexual partner simultaneously is because during caregiving activities physical contact is no longer necessarily sexual. It can be hard to turn on and off sexual reactions at will. For most of our marital lives, touch was at least affectionate and sensual, if not actually sexual. It now becomes more clinical and may even be embarrassing or pain-producing. Some couples manage to retain the sexual overtones implicit in bathing and dressing activities, but most have difficulty feeling the same sexual spark when it comes to changing the sheets, feeding, giving wound care, or helping with toileting.

These challenges are not unique to people facing end-stage cancer. For example, couples in which one has suffered paralysis from a stroke or a spinal cord injury also face these obstacles. Whenever possible, such couples should try to find alternative ways of meeting caregiving needs. If a third person can take over those tasks, the spouse can retain more of the marital roles, promoting a healthier sexual relationship. If use of a separate caregiver isn't possible, partners must discuss this challenge frankly. Some solutions include setting aside a special place just for sex, and not using that bed for sleeping or convalescing. Some spouses separate the roles by literally taking off the gloves; during caregiving activities they wear latex gloves for better sanitation and easier cleanup, but during sex they leave themselves fully exposed. Some people choose a particular time of day for sex and mentally switch gears into the sexual mode. It's absolutely possible to continue a sexual relationship in these circumstances if you open your mind to it. Remember, nurses have fallen in love with patients in spite of strict regulations against pursuing such entanglements!

Risks for Sexual Dysfunctions

The effect of pain.   Usually cancer does not itself physically alter normal sexual function unless it continues to grow unchecked and starts impinging on nerve and blood vessel function. When difficulties arise in loss of sex drive, painful intercourse, erectile problems, and other sexual obstacles, it's usually because of treatments, fatigue, or the psychological trauma of the disease.

The one exception to this is pain from advanced cancer or as a complication of a treatment. Chronic pain from any cause can contribute to sexual dysfunction in both women and men because it interferes with concentration, relaxation, and enjoyment. It occasionally leads to low sexual desire, the inability to reach orgasm, or erectile difficulty.

One way to reduce the pain of cancer is to take a prescribed pain-relieving medication thirty to sixty minutes before starting sexual activity. If pain persists and becomes a serious distraction, ask your doctor for a stronger prescription or a different medication. (Be aware that narcotic pain relievers can decrease sexual response.) Sometimes new intercourse positions and use of pillows to support various parts help as well. A heating pad, a hot water bottle, or a massage can help occasionally. More aggressive steps may be necessary for treating intractable pain associated with advanced cancer, such as chemotherapy or surgically cutting nerves that transmit pain sensations.

Emotions that block sexual performance.   Not only do the feelings of guilt, anger, depression, shame, or fear emerge when cancer first appears, but they also surface whenever treatments don't go as expected, side effects exasperate, cancer recurs, or just for no apparent reason. Strong emotions can inhibit sexual arousal. Unless you're one of the few people who can block them out and find that sex is a helpful distraction from your problems, it may be best not to try to have sex whenever emotions are intense and to wait a few hours. If emotions continually interfere with sexual enjoyment, it's time to get professional counseling.

Spectatoring.   Some cancer patients obsessively monitor everything about their bodies, watching for signs of advancing disease or side effects of treatments. If they watch too closely for changes during sex, this constitutes "spectatoring" (see chapters 4 and 5 for help). Spectatoring can block the body's ability to become aroused or have an orgasm. While heightened sensitivity to physical well-being is understandable when a person's health is in jeopardy, it's important to let go of those concerns occasionally so we can experience pleasure as well.

Withdrawal from physical contact.   Many people with cancer have a suddenly exceptional need for more privacy than usual. Not only does cancer upset our balance and sense of well-being, but also the health care system and cancer treatments can leave us feeling dehumanized. Frequent examinations and procedures performed on our bodies feel like such an invasion and violation of our personal space and dignity that the cumulative effect is psychologically similar to rape.

The stress of enduring so much touching and looking at our bodies by health care providers (even though they are trying to help us) and the loss of control over our normal routines can lead to withdrawal from human contact. We just want to be left alone sometimes. When our spouses try to give us a shoulder rub, we find ourselves shrinking away. We can't bear the thought of sex right now. We don't want to be touched.

Unless we can analyze and share our reactions, our actions may come across as a rejection of sex or the partner. Fortunately, these feelings are temporary, but in the meantime we're likely to feel guilty and our spouses are going to feel hurt. The solution for this problem and others that inevitably creep up throughout the course of cancer is to *talk, talk, talk!* Don't pull into your shell and isolate yourself. You and your spouse need to express your feelings to each other often without judging harshly. Just accept the feelings as valid and discuss what to do to improve the situation.

> *When Theo had to have his pancreas removed for cancer, the surgical wound got infected. For a while we had a Registered Nurse come to the house to give him antibiotics and change the dressings. He got really touchy whenever she came. He would never let me stick around to help or just be friendly. He got real short-tempered, too, and wouldn't let me touch him. One day I managed to pull the nurse aside as she was leaving and started asking questions. Apparently his wound had pulled open and was draining a lot of pus or something. He was really embarrassed and didn't want me to know or see him like that. We'd always talked about everything, so this really hurt my feelings. I couldn't forget about it, so I just straight out told him I knew what was going on and asked him why he hadn't told me. He admitted he knew it was silly to feel embarrassed, but he'd always been the strong one and felt like he was letting me down with all the health problems. We talked and talked. It was like a dam broke. I still didn't insist on*

watching his dressing changes, but after that we never had any more secrets from each other—no matter how ridiculous they seemed.

A sense of humor is an important way of coping. Look at cancer as a challenge to be conquered with grace and adventure. Find the silly moments among the struggles. Laugh at the absurdities. If your ostomy bag leaks, keep your cool and threaten to switch to sandwich bags. Give your surgical scar a funny nickname. Laughter lifts your spirit, improves circulation, expands the lungs, and boosts the immune system. Remember, what makes you sexually attractive has more to do with your attitude than anything else.

HOW CANCER TREATMENTS AFFECT SEXUALITY

In spite of the recent boon in research and the development of new drugs to slow the cancer growth, we still use three primary methods of treatment: surgery, radiation, and chemotherapy, alone or in combination. Each therapy has implications for sexuality, both in the immediate treatment period and in the long term. It has at times seemed that the treatments are worse than the cancer. The choice, though, is to let cancer take its course or learn how to cope with the treatments and continue living life as fully as possible. Living a full life includes maximizing sexual potential—usually in new ways.

Surgery to Treat Cancer

Start by scheduling a visit with a member of a support group dealing with your particular condition, preferably while you're still in the hospital. This contact will do wonders for you by giving hope and supplying practical information on how to adjust. This person can be a role model for you. He or she can probably supply phone numbers or addresses of companies specializing in products for your particular needs. Also ask hospital personnel if there is a nurse on staff who specializes in postoperative patient education.

The products you may need include special undergarments, artificial breasts to make your clothing fit better, appliances for your colostomy, prosthetics for amputated limbs, or other items. Taking steps immediately after surgery to make your appearance as pleasing as possible will improve your feelings about yourself. Investigate reconstructive surgery, such as formation of a new breast using an artificial implant or tissue from other parts of your body. Reconstructive surgery doesn't necessarily prevent a sexual dysfunction, but it can improve self-esteem and restore feelings of control over your situation. Some physicians offer reconstruction as part of the same procedure to remove the cancer, rather than splitting the operation into parts several weeks or months later.

Another difficult, but necessary, step is to look at your incision, then allow your spouse to see it. Most people are pleasantly surprised because the incision doesn't look as bad as they had feared. Spouses must realize that their reaction at the first sight of the surgical scar is extremely critical, that they can greatly influence your feelings of self-esteem and your attitude toward sex. They should plan how to react and try to have a positive expression. Spouses who avoid looking at or touching the scar during sex may inadvertently send negative messages of aversion, but may instead just be trying to preserve your feelings, particularly if you seem self-conscious about it.

No one expects your spouse to be insincere or grimly cheerful. However, he or she needs to express love, acceptance, and sympathy for what you are going through, comment on how fine a job the surgeon did to make your incision look good, and assure you it will look even better in a few weeks.

Resume intercourse as soon as possible after surgery, especially if you're going to have radiation therapy next. Not only will radiation introduce new side effects that can disrupt sex, but also partners should interrupt sexual activity for as short a period as possible to avoid sexual distancing that strains the relationship. Intercourse is also beneficial for the woman facing pelvic radiation because it helps maintain the patency of her vagina. For both men and women, sexual activity promotes healing in the abdomen and pelvis by increasing circulation.

Okay, I'll confess. I cried the first time we started having sex again after my surgery. It wasn't because I felt anxious or had any serious pain. It was because I had missed it so much. For the past ten years or so I had thought sex was something I could take or leave, until I had to leave it for a while. When Bart and I made love again, it felt like I had just come through a desert alone and he was rescuing me. Even though we hadn't been apart, I still missed him. I missed the sharing of our most private activity and the warmth and the smell of him after sex and everything else about it. Having cancer has taught me a lot about myself and my need for sex.

You may have some anxiety about how intercourse will feel the first time after surgery. Ideally, intercourse shouldn't be part of your first postoperative sexual encounter, though. Even before the surgical site has finished healing, you can begin sexual stimulation to orgasm without intercourse. One of the best ways to boost confidence is to have an orgasm alone. It helps overcome fears about pain and lets you learn how your body *may* function differently now.

If you had surgery in the abdomen or the pelvis, differences you may notice are due to the cutting or removal of lymph nodes, ligaments, blood vessels, nerves, or other tissues that play a role in sexuality. There may be some loss of sensation or decreased engorgement in the genitals. These changes are not necessarily permanent, however. Because of the trauma of surgery and the swelling of tissues, pressure on nerves and blood vessels can inhibit normal function for as long as six months. Let's look at specific types of surgical treatments and how each impacts on sexuality.

Testicular cancer. Most cases of testicular cancer occur in men under age forty. Regardless of age, though, surgical removal of the affected testis is absolutely necessary. If the cosmetic appearance of the scrotum is important, implantation of an artificial testis is possible. As long as one testis remains, sperm production and testosterone levels remain adequate. In rare cases necessitating removal of both testes, testosterone replacement therapy (TRT) is important for maintenance of the sex drive, erections, and male physical characteristics. However, TRT is not an option if cancer continues or is of the type that testosterone stimulates. If testicular cancer is advanced and more of the tissue around the reproductive organs must be excised, ejaculatory fluid volume may decrease due to lymph node removal. Nerve damage may also cause retrograde ejaculation, in which sperm flow into the bladder rather than out through the penis. These "dry orgasms" are still pleasurable but ineffective for fertility.

Cervical or uterine cancer.   A woman who has a hysterectomy for cancer may have ligaments, ovaries, and lymph nodes removed in addition to the uterus to better assure eradication of all affected tissues. The more extensive the surgery, the more likely is nerve or blood vessel damage, leading to diminished engorgement or pelvic and genital numbness. It is quite normal for pelvic tissues to swell for a while after surgery, affecting circulation and function, so wait several weeks before concluding that a change is permanent.

Engorgement is not necessary for sexual function, but arousal does feel different. Furthermore, without engorgement of the vagina less moisture can seep through the vaginal wall for lubrication. Use an artificial lubricant to reduce friction and pain during intercourse.

Permanent numbness of the genitals, particularly the clitoris, caused when surgery damages nerves is more disturbing. Science can't yet reverse nerve loss. Therefore, if it's more difficult to feel adequate stimulation of the clitoris, the stimulation must become more intense. An excellent option is to use a vibrator or a hand-held shower nozzle with adjustable spray strengths for just the right intensity of clitoral stimulation. Be careful about stimulating too vigorously. Inspect your genitals using a mirror to see if redness persists an hour after orgasm or if there has been any bruising or skin irritation. Diabetic women especially must take care to avoid tissue damage because healing takes longer.

> *I used to think vibrators were something used only by kinky people or lonely women who couldn't attract a man. I'll be forever grateful to the gal in my book club who disclosed to us that she and her husband had used a vibrator for years to give her the boost she needed (apparently she'd had some operation that left her "dead down there," as she put it). When I needed the same help, I dialed her up and she let me borrow her catalog so I could order one. Since then, I've found that the electric massagers at the drugstore work great, too, but some of them are too noisy, so you have to shop around.*

Cystectomy for bladder cancer.   For men, total bladder removal (a radical cystectomy) causes permanent loss of erections unless the surgeon uses nerve-sparing techniques, isolating nerves responsible for sexual function and taking care not to cut them when removing cancerous tissues. Another risk is the possibility of severing blood vessels to the corpora cavernosa, causing permanent loss of erections. Several options to artificially restore erections are described in chapter 4. If nerve-sparing surgery succeeds, a man will probably still be able to have orgasms with or without natural or artificially produced erections. Erections are not necessary for orgasm, only intercourse.

A woman who undergoes a radical cystectomy usually has more removed than just the bladder. A complete hysterectomy and oophorectomy (removal of the ovaries) are not unusual. A cystectomy also involves removal of part of the front of the vaginal wall near the bladder. Vaginal repair is necessary, often leaving it somewhat shorter and narrower at the top. Dyspareunia (painful intercourse) may also be due to loss of the ovaries affecting lubrication and sex drive. Refer to chapter 6 for much more information about how to adjust to a hysterectomy or oophorectomy. About two to three weeks after the surgery, when her incision has sealed sufficiently, the woman can start reestablishing sexual function by using a vaginal dilator or dildo while alone to test the space limits of her vagina. She should begin with a small size, gradually increasing over a period of days or weeks to one about the size of an erect penis. She must teach her husband how deeply he can now penetrate without causing pain. Undoubtedly she will prefer intercourse positions that prevent deep penile penetration.

The good news about a radical cystectomy is that most women don't lose their ability to have orgasms. They may notice decreased engorgement if surgery removed or cut blood vessels, though, perhaps diminishing vaginal lubrication.

Bone cancer.   Amputation of the affected limb is necessary for treatment of cancer that originates in the bone of an arm or leg. Cancer that has spread to the bone from another site may or may not be treated surgically. In those cases, radiation or chemotherapy are more common treatments.

Amputation presents a variety of sexual problems: difficulty getting into certain positions and holding them for sexual activities, pain sensed in the affected limb—even after its removal and the scar has healed ("phantom" limb pain), and the psychological impact of losing an arm or a leg. It is your choice whether to replace your missing limb with a prosthesis, but most people find that doing so not only helps with equilibrium and support, it also boosts feelings of sexual attractiveness and promotes a more natural appearance. Wearing the prosthesis during sex will help you keep your balance better and make it easier to maintain a position. Talk to others who have gone through your same experience, asking for tips on how to prevent rashes and perspiration under the prosthesis, ways to wear clothing that present a more natural appearance, and how to prevent embarrassing sounds or slippage. Solving problems common to prosthesis wearers will decrease your self-consciousness during sexual activity.

Sexual activity seems to provoke phantom limb pain. We don't fully understand why, except that the entire body experiences heightened nervous tension during sexual arousal. Experiment with various techniques to find one that works best to help you overcome or adapt to this problem. Suggestions include massaging the stump, taking a pain reliever thirty minutes before sexual activity, or applying a heating pad, ice bag, or anesthetic ointment to the stump. Some people claim one alcoholic drink before sex reduces phantom limb pain, but alcohol can also reduce sexual responsiveness. Another suggestion worth a try is to massage and scratch the remaining limb on your *other* side, targeting the same area where the phantom pain is worst.

Cancer of the penis.   Cancer of the penis is such a frightening prospect that the few (almost always uncircumcised) men who fall prey to it often delay finding out what is wrong. By detecting penile cancer early, though, a surgeon can usually leave most of the penis intact and functional, removing only the affected portion. If, however, cancer has progressed to where removal of the end of the penis is necessary, the surgeon will create a new opening at the end of the penile stump for urination and ejaculation. The stump can still become erect during sexual arousal. Even though the sensitive tip of the penis is no longer there, orgasms are still possible, although intercourse depends on the new length of the penis. Through stimulation of the penile stump, the nipples, the perineum (the area behind the scrotum), the scrotum, the anal area, the ears, and other erogenous zones, a man can relearn to orgasm quite satisfactorily.

With a total penectomy (removal of the entire penis), the surgeon leaves an opening for urination and ejaculation that sits fairly flush with the front of the abdomen where the penis used to be. Even men who've had a penectomy can learn to orgasm through stimulation of the newly created opening and other erogenous body parts. There are two options for intercourse: (1) a dildo to simulate intercourse or (2) cosmetic surgery to form a new penis using other body tissues, along with a penile implant to produce an erection. The key here, as with all of these conditions, is for couples to experiment and discuss sexual matters to find what remaining potential they have and to take advantage of what science has to offer.

> *I've been through everything. I "lost" my penis to cancer more than fifteen years ago, when I was only fifty-two, so you can believe me when I say that sex is possible no matter what. Of course, my wife deserves some credit, too. We started playing around one night about six months after the operation. I can't even remember how we got started, but one thing led to another and she made it clear that she wanted me bad! I played with her and put my fingers inside and she came in no time, but wouldn't stop. She had her hands all over my body and excited me in ways I thought required a penis. I was hot and really shocked to discover that I wanted sex as much as ever. We kept trying new stuff over the next several weeks and soon I was having orgasms again— ejaculating through my pee hole and everything! My favorite technique is for her to lightly rub my pee hole with Vaseline and tongue my ears while I touch her all over, too.*

Colostomy, iliostomy, or urostomy. Sometimes treatment of colon, intestinal, or urinary tract cancer or other conditions necessitates removal of a portion of the lower intestine (colostomy), small intestine (iliostomy), or rerouting of urine (urostomy) because the surgeon cannot sew the remaining healthy tissue ends together. A stoma or "ostomy" is an artificially created orifice through which waste products pass to the outside, rather than being urinated or defecated normally. Although some people with a colostomy get by with occasionally wearing a simple pad over the stoma, most ostomates must always wear a collection bag called an "appliance." The appliance sticks to the skin around the opening with the aid of special adhesives.

Several concerns arise for the wearer of an appliance, such as worrying if other people can see it through clothing, anxiety that the bag will dislodge or spill open, fear that others can smell bad odors from the bag, or uneasiness about passing gas from the intestine that will make noise or inflate the bag. These anxieties arouse old childhood feelings of shame we learned from our parents when we had an accident and soiled our clothing. There are excellent resources for learning how to prevent problems. Support groups and ostomy nurses can teach you how to affix the appliance so it won't slip or spill open.

One unnecessary worry people with an ostomy have is that they might harm it during sex. The stoma is quite resilient, though. Another worry is that it will disgust the partner. If you would rather your spouse not see your collection bag during sex, cover it up. Women can wear a garter belt or crotchless panties. Either gender can wear a top that comes down over the area or a tube wrap to keep the bag from being jostled. A man can purchase an extra-wide jock strap, cut off the leggings, and tuck the appliance under the waistband during sex. He could buy a striking cummerbund and "dress up" for sex.

Empty your bag before sex so it will lie flat. Don't eat or drink an hour before sex either, because that stimulates intestinal and kidney activity. Use intercourse positions that don't put weight on the pouch unless you've secured it well underneath a snug garment or wrap. Also avoid positions that make the appliance slide back and forth.

You may find that it is sexually arousing to stimulate the stoma. Some people even have orgasms that way. This is acceptable as long as you don't traumatize it. Never use the stoma for intercourse. Don't put anything into it, because the inside lining is fragile and easily torn. Furthermore, germs inside the intestine can infect the penis.

Don't be too secretive about your ostomy around your spouse. As with a surgical scar, your spouse will see it eventually and will probably say that it's not nearly as offensive or as big a deal as expected.

If you had a complete excision of your rectum or colon to remove cancer, you may have additional sexual challenges. For men, erectile difficulty may result from nerve or blood vessel damage from surgery in the pelvis. This was much more of a problem in the past with "abdominal perineal resections" in which the surgeon reached the colon by cutting behind the scrotum, severing important nerves in the process. With better surgical techniques, permanent erectile loss is not as likely. If it does happen, though, review chapter 4 for ways to reestablish erections. Women sometimes have temporary dyspareunia after a colectomy (colon removal) due to trauma in the pelvic area. They should see a physician about intercourse pain persisting longer than three months.

Breast cancer.   The breast is currently an important sexual symbol (just look at all the interest in push-up bras and breast implants). Surgical removal of a breast (mastectomy) can severely alter a woman's impression of herself as a sexual and feminine being. Its loss also affects her as a violation of her personal space, especially her physical sexual self. Even if done for the right reasons by a caring surgeon, a mastectomy can still leave a woman feeling as emotionally damaged as a sexual assault.

Reconstruction of a new breast surgically, or obtaining a breast prosthesis as soon as possible, renews self-worth. A woman can wear a prosthesis within a couple of days after surgery so that clothing fits better and she can feel better about her appearance. She must, however, still come to terms with the alteration of her physical appearance. This is accomplished through counseling, discussing feelings with others who've had mastectomies, and witnessing the accepting attitude of her husband. He can help her regain self-respect and feelings of femininity by praising her efforts to look nice. He should compliment her and tell her how pretty and sexy she is. He must affirm his love for her no matter what, and convince her that he is in love with her, not her breasts. Something as simple as reaching for her hand or kissing her spontaneously means so much.

A mastectomy doesn't physically change genital function, sex drive, or the ability to orgasm. Any decrease in sex drive lasting more than a few weeks is undoubtedly due to the psychological impact of cancer or the surgery. However, a mastectomy does have other physical implications for sex. Removal of muscles in the chest and shoulder can hamper certain positions. She should avoid sexual positions that put pressure on her affected arm or require it to support weight. Surgery can leave a woman's arm on her affected side quite swollen for several weeks or even months, particularly if she had lymph nodes removed. In addition, post-surgical pain can interfere with her ability to relax or enjoy sex. A nonprescription pain reliever thirty to sixty minutes before starting sexual activity will help reduce the distraction of pain.

I had to wear an elastic wrap bandage around my arm for quite a while after my mastectomy, because they took out so many lymph nodes, causing fluid to collect in my arm. This meant that even though I was wearing a mastectomy bra and looked like I still had a breast, everyone could see my arm and asked what was wrong. I finally learned to have a short standard answer ready because, not only was it embarrassing to me, but also the people I was talking to usually got "deer in the headlights" looks on their faces when they started to hear my explanation. While the arm hurt and ached, it didn't really bother me except during sex. It was awfully hard to get comfortable and still be in a position where sex was possible. I bought a bunch of pillows and propped my arm up on them. We got by until gradually the pain and swelling let up.

A good position for intercourse is side-lying, in which the woman lies on her better side with her back to her husband. By curling her knees up toward her chest, moving her upper body away from him, resting her affected arm on pillows in front of her, and "presenting" her genitals by tilting her pelvis back toward him, intercourse from behind is easily possible without using her sore arm or contacting the mastectomy site.

Cancer of the lungs or neck area.   With removal of a portion or all of a lung, the biggest challenges to sexual function are decreased respiratory capacity and fatigue. Many people find they can no longer breathe comfortably while lying flat in bed. They must adapt their position during intercourse to allow them to sit more upright. Some people think that by lying on the side of their affected lung, their healthy lung can expand better. Others find that lying on the side of the healthy lung takes pressure off the affected side and reduces pain, so experiment to find what works better for you.

With both neck and lung surgery, an unexpected distraction is that as sexual tension builds, breathing becomes noisier and more rapid. Faster, deeper breathing loosens respiratory secretions, possibly stimulating a coughing spell. It becomes necessary to stop and cough a while to clear out the congestion before continuing—if there's enough strength left to continue. Therefore it's better to have sex after first clearing secretions. Since it takes a couple of hours upon awakening to dislodge secretions that build up during the night, sex in the late morning or early afternoon is usually better while the day is still young enough for fatigue to be less of a problem. Even then, it takes an understanding spouse not to give up on sex in frustration when coughing spells hit, but to be patient and encouraging.

Surgery on the neck for cancer of the larynx (voice box), pharynx (throat), or mouth can cause breathing problems, but also alters appearance. If it's necessary to remove a portion of the neck, jaw, cheek, or lip to excise the cancer, the result can be disfiguring. Although cosmetic surgery is possible, total restoration is unlikely. Self-respect and feelings of being sexually attractive depend on a person's inner strength and the attitude of the spouse. A partner who continues to express love and sexual interest can make all the difference in the affected person's desire for sex.

Special problems these people have also include difficulty eating and talking. Sometimes the ability to speak is lost entirely, making communication much more difficult. An electrolarynx (a mechanical device held up to the neck to transmit audible vibrations that sound like a robotic voice) or learning how to use esophageal air to belch words can reestablish a type of audible speech that's certainly faster than handwritten messages and easier to hear than whispers. It's difficult to control volume and decreases the range of voice inflections, though. The subtleties lost may make sexual communication seem unemotional or harsh when that's not the speaker's intent at all. The spouse needs to understand this and read the nonverbal behaviors and facial expressions to interpret the speech correctly. Even if the voice box remains intact, surgery around it can change voice quality or decrease volume, making communication more difficult, too.

Sometimes a tracheostomy (a hole in the front of the neck through which to breathe) is necessary. The spouse may worry about inadvertently suffocating the partner during sex by accidentally covering the tracheostomy or dislodging the device that keeps it open. Be assured that nurses teach how to take care of a tracheostomy before hospital dismissal or arrange for home health care. As long as a person is conscious, he or she will struggle if the airway becomes blocked, so suffocation is not likely anyway.

One complaint about many people who've had a tracheostomy is that they lose their sense of smell. They may not be aware of bad body odors, making it more difficult for their partners to find them sexually attractive. Rigorous attention to personal hygiene and good dental care must continue to avoid offending anyone.

Pelvic exenteration.   Pelvic exenteration is used most often in women whose cancer has spread throughout their pelvic organs. It involves a complete hysterectomy and oophorectomy, removal of most or all of the vagina, and possibly removal of the bladder and rectum. Obviously, the sexual implications are great. Not only is there loss of estrogen and testosterone and probable severing of sexual nerves and blood vessels, but also, with removal of the vagina, intercourse becomes impossible. If desired, a woman can have vaginal reconstruction at the same time as her pelvic exenteration or wait. The surgeon will create a vaginalike passageway that permits shallow intercourse. After removal of the vagina, some women report phantom vaginal sensations, just as a person who's had an amputation can sometimes still sense the missing leg.

Most women who've had pelvic exenteration discontinue all sexual activity. This isn't surprising in light of the extensive disruption of normal genital function, the pain of such extensive surgery, and the psychological impact. However, sex is still possible. A woman can maximize her potential by experimenting with the genital sensations she still has. She might have enough nerve function to reach orgasm through stimulation of the clitoris. She can get more intense stimulation from a vibrator. She can learn to orgasm through nipple stimulation. She can provide sexual stimulation to her husband by using oral and manual techniques, making herself available for intercourse between the breasts, between the thighs, and other variations. The important factor here is openness to experimentation, allowing sex to grow into new dimensions.

Cancer on the vulva.   A vulvectomy is surgical removal of the labial skin folds, clitoris, and perhaps the vagina. Since nerves leading to the clitoral area remain intact, it's possible to retain orgasmic ability. The remaining tissue around the area where the clitoris used to be can be massaged once the surgical scar has healed. In conjunction with nipple stimulation this can be a satisfactory compromise, permitting a great deal of sexual satisfaction. If vaginal intercourse remains possible, the woman still has a full range of internal erotic sensations as well.

A vulvectomy leaves the urinary opening just inside the vagina in a more exposed position than before. If the vagina remains intact, intercourse may cause it to become sore more easily. Solutions include use of artificial lubricant and changing intercourse positions to find one that changes the angle of entry.

Radiation Therapy to Treat Cancer

Radiation therapy can be a valuable way to stop the growth of several forms of cancer. The energy waves are more lethal to cells while they are dividing, and cancer cells divide more often than normal cells. Some normal cells are more vulnerable to the effects of radiation, too, especially those with a faster metabolism, such as hair roots and the testes. Delicate tissues lining various organ tracts (such as the intestines, urinary system, and genitals) are also more susceptible.

Most radiation is administered by directing a beam from outside the body toward the cancer. For some forms of cancer, though (e.g., cervical, thyroid, uterine, or prostate cancer), the physician can position radioactive "seeds" or pellets directly inside the affected organ. The radioactive range of some pellets is less than an inch, pose no threat to others (even during intercourse), and may be left in permanently. Other types are potent even to other people who come within a few feet and must be removed after a few days. If you have the latter type, you will remain hospitalized and may only have nonpregnant visitors more than eighteen years old for a few minutes each day, if they stay at least six feet away. This form of radiation affects sexuality more in the short term by temporarily disrupting physical contact with the spouse. Those few days can seem to take forever and require special patience.

Brachytherapy is another way of delivering a high dose of internal radiation, through tubes directed to the target organ from the outside for a few minutes each treatment. This method doesn't require hospitalization, and the patient poses no radiation risk to others.

The side effects of internal radiation are similar to those for external radiation, except that external beam radiation also affects the skin over the surface of the targeted area. Problems should reduce in severity as the treatments stop, but not always. Sometimes they become more troublesome and last a few months. Regardless of the radiation method, sexuality can be affected. Let's review how.

Skin problems with external beam radiation.   Within two to three weeks after treatments start, the skin may look sunburned, dry, and flaky. Resist the impulse to scratch if it becomes itchy. Continue to bathe daily but stop using soap, lotions, scented powder, or medications on the area for a while (a little baby powder or mineral oil is all right). Protect the area from the sun. Don't expose it to heat or cold, not even a hot water bottle, heating pad, or ice bag. Wear loose-fitting clothing, choosing cotton and "breathable" fabrics instead of synthetics. Expect the hair on the skin in the radiated area to fall out, but to regrow later.

Sometimes oncologists draw lines on the skin to mark the target area for radiation. Leave the lines there. Understandably, they're not attractive and may mar the aesthetic affect of nudity and detract from your feelings of sexiness. Their importance overrides the temporary inconvenience, though.

> *I hated those lines they drew on me for my radiation treatments. I had always scolded my kids for drawing on themselves, and I absolutely hate tattoos. Those lines just served to disrupt my mood during sex because they were a reminder that I had cancer. I found them to be so disturbing that I had sex only when I could cover them with clothing or could have sex in the dark.*

Bowel problems.   Radiation of the abdomen or pelvis usually irritates the intestines, particularly the colon. To prevent constipation, take a "stool softener" every day, such as Colace (docusate sodium), but not laxatives, which can irritate the bowels further and cause bleeding. More likely your problem will be diarrhea, not constipation. Drink at least eight full glasses of beverages every day and switch to a diet with little waste residue or fiber. Keep your rectal area well cleansed and dry to avoid erosion caused by the acidic diarrhea.

Report any problems to your physician or nurse to obtain medications to reduce discomfort and for suggestions on other ways to become more comfortable. Unfortunately, information on how radiation affects the genitals and reproductive tract is harder to find, so let's examine these problems in detail.

Sexual problems in men (see also chapter 7 regarding prostate cancer).   Erectile problems occur at least temporarily in up to half of all men receiving radiation, usually because radiation irritates nerves that produce erections. Sometimes irritation shows up as a small amount of blood in the ejaculate fluid. This bleeding is short-lived and may not even be visible to the naked eye.

Sperm production can also decline or cease. Some sperm take on abnormal shapes, even with low doses of radiation. Testosterone can drop, too, causing loss of sex drive and erections. Generally, once therapy stops, sperm and testosterone production returns to normal. Sperm shapes may continue to be abnormal, however, sometimes permanently. Even if the sperm look normal, the DNA inside may not be.

This is a difficult issue for men who want to continue to father children. Even average radiation doses can permanently damage part of the testes. Wait at least a year or two after radiation to father a child to let the testes recover. Even better, though, is to bank your sperm for later use before undergoing radiation. In some cancer cases, such as Hodgkin's disease or lymphoma, it may be possible for your physician to shield your testes with lead to reduce their exposure.

Sexual problems in women.   Radiation of the abdomen, pelvis, or fragile genital tissues can cause fibrosity and loss of elasticity, making engorgement more difficult. Most women lose their pubic hair. While the hair will regrow after therapy stops, the fibrosis is permanent. Before the vaginal wall becomes fibrotic, though, it first passes through a period when the tissues ("mucosa") are so delicate that intercourse can cause tiny cracks in the surface. Intercourse must be slow and gentle. Lubrication of the vagina with one of the many nonprescription products available is very important. Stop having intercourse for a few days if the pain becomes severe, but don't delay resumption longer than necessary.

The next stage is fibrosis, causing vaginal shortening and narrowing. Fibrosis is similar to scar tissue, which doesn't stretch as well as normal tissue. The wise woman will keep her vagina as healthy as possible during radiation therapy by continuing to have intercourse, if allowed. External-beam radiation doesn't make the woman radioactive or dangerous to touch, so there should be no limitations in such cases.

If radiation pellets are *implanted* temporarily, though, intercourse may be forbidden for a while. In the meantime the woman should insert a dildo or vaginal dilator at least every other day for fifteen minutes to stretch the vaginal walls. As soon as the surgeon removes the implants, the couple should resume intercourse before fibrosis fully develops. This helps the couple stay close and preserves the vagina, keeping it free of adhesions and preventing loss of its capacity for expansion. Frequent orgasms are important, too, to nourish the vagina with greater blood flow.

If fibrosis has already started in your vagina, you can still restore much of its resilience. Purchase a set of vaginal dilators from a medical supply company or fashion your own using clean, nontoxic, smooth, tube-shaped objects that are closed and rounded at the tip. Start with one about half an inch in diameter. Lubricate it well, slowly slide it into the vagina, and leave it there for fifteen minutes. Repeat at least one to three times a day, moving to the next larger size when you have no pain until you can comfortably insert one about the size of your husband's erect penis. You should now be able to have intercourse without difficulty. If not, see your family physician or gynecologist for a vaginal examination.

Some women who have radiation discover that semen burns. Until the genitals recover, the husband can wear a condom or practice coitus interruptus (withdrawing the penis from the vagina just before ejaculation). This problem is not an adequate reason for discontinuing intercourse, though. Intercourse is so important to vaginal health that a couple should do whatever is necessary to relieve any pain so the woman doesn't become tense in anticipation of it.

A premenopausal woman who still has her ovaries will probably experience ovarian shutdown during radiation. Resulting estrogen deficiency is temporary, but does require management through use of artificial lubricants on and in the genitals. The physician probably won't prescribe estrogen replacement because it makes some tumors grow more rapidly.

Sometimes radiation for Hodgkin's disease or lymphoma causes the ovaries to shrink and stop functioning permanently. This renders a younger woman sterile and brings on premature menopause. The physician may be able to shield the ovaries from radiation by placing a lead barrier around them, or surgically move them to a new position in the abdomen away from radiation.

The wisdom of becoming pregnant after radiation is questionable due to possible genetic damage to the ova (eggs). While men produce new sperm throughout life, women don't make new ova. All the ova they will ever have reside in the ovaries from birth. If radiation harms them, there is no possibility for making new normal ones. Ova can possibly be extracted and frozen prior to radiation if a woman wants to leave later pregnancy open as an option.

If the cervix isn't removed by a hysterectomy, vigorous intercourse can irritate it, making vaginal secretions look pink-tinged with blood. Rather than avoiding deep penile penetration altogether (because it helps prevent vaginal fibrosis), these women just shouldn't bounce or thrust sharply during intercourse until tissues return to normal after radiation therapy.

Chemotherapy

Chemotherapy is a broad category of medications and chemicals that usually act against cancer by producing toxic effects on the rapidly growing cancer cells. These medications enter the bloodstream and don't just stay in the area where the cancer is, even if the "first pass" is from an injection into the artery supplying the cancer. Therefore, the whole body is vulnerable to side effects, making sexual problems pretty much the same and predictable from one person to the next regardless of whether the cancer is in the breast, bone, brain, blood, or elsewhere.

Because chemotherapeutic agents are more toxic to cells with a high metabolism and a rapid rate of growth, some normal body cells are also at risk: hair roots, the testes and ovaries, the lining of the intestinal tract, the bone marrow that makes blood cells and platelets, and so forth. Mucosal membranes, such as the lining of the mouth, the urinary tract, and the vagina, also have more problems. Blood may appear in the urine, not only because of bladder and urinary passageway irritation, but also, with fewer blood platelets in circulation, bleeding doesn't stop as quickly. Some chemotherapeutic agents cause fibrosis in the kidneys, lungs, and liver, or can damage the heart.

Chemotherapy is not new, but we are getting better at controlling some serious side effects. Rather than analyze each chemotherapeutic agent for sexual implications, let's examine chemotherapy as a whole and identify how to overcome or adapt to sexual problems.

Fatigue.   Insomnia due to worry about cancer may contribute to fatigue, but chemotherapy is likely to cause anemia, the reduction of red blood cells that carry oxygen throughout the body that also leaves a person weak and tired. Chemotherapy can destroy bone marrow where new red blood cells are made. Sometimes this type of anemia is a side effect of treatment, but at other times it is intentional, as in the case of leukemia or lymphoma, because it stops new cancerous blood cells from forming.

Anemia from chemotherapy may also result from excessive bleeding anywhere in the body, because the marrow also produces white blood cells and platelets. Platelets help blood to clot when we bleed. Signs of low quantities of platelets include nosebleeds, bleeding gums, bruising easily, and rectal bleeding with bowel movements.

Regardless of whether your anemia stems from bleeding or diminished red blood cell production, you will tire easily and have little energy for even routine activities. Tell your physician if fatigue becomes severe. After chemotherapy stops, the blood does rebuild and fatigue gradually disappears.

In special cases it's necessary to totally destroy the bone marrow to eradicate certain cancers. New marrow obtained by transplant from a donor then begins building new normal blood. A variation of this is peripheral blood stem cell transplantation, in which the person with cancer donates his or her own blood in advance of chemotherapy. The blood is then treated and prepared for reinfusion. In the meantime, very high doses of chemotherapy or radiation effectively kill the cancer within the bone marrow. The stem cells (precursor cells from which blood is formed) are then placed back into the body to form new, healthy cells. Hospitalization lasts one to two months, but full recovery of strength can take a year.

Sexuality is seriously disrupted by this type of therapy. During hospitalization protective isolation from contact with people not wearing germ-free coverings is critically important because the number of white blood cells to fight infection is very low. Visits are discouraged. Even spouses may stay only briefly. Fatigue is extreme. Sex is not very important under these circumstances, but the need for spousal support is profound. Feelings of loneliness and fear can be overwhelming. The couple must find new ways to communicate love during this time. The healthy spouse must also be allowed to meet sexual needs alone without guilt.

Fortunately, chemotherapy is not nearly so difficult for most people, but you may still battle fatigue. If you experience considerable weakness during your therapy, you, too, will probably have less interest in sex. The body protects itself by conserving energy. Or perhaps you still have a strong sex drive but just can't muster the energy to act. If your husband or wife wants sex but you're too exhausted, use less demanding sexual techniques. Choose positions that don't require you to bear weight or perform much thrusting. Have sex when you're most rested. Build an afternoon nap into your schedule, then have sex upon awakening.

> *I felt so worn out during part of my chemotherapy that I couldn't even get up the strength to wiggle a little during sex. At that point I didn't care if I ever had sex again (that feeling didn't last—thank God!). I told Francine that I was willing just to hold her and be there while she took care of herself. In that way she could feel like we were still being intimate. She was a little self-conscious at first, but relaxed after a while. She even admitted to me later that playing with herself in front of me had been one of her secret sex fantasies. I just refused to let myself feel guilty about being unable to meet all of her sexual needs during that time. At least she wasn't turning to someone else!*

Feelings of guilt about what we truly can't do are unproductive. Look at this particular challenge as an inconvenience, not something that indicates a failure on your part.

Mouth and intestinal problems. Stomatitis (inflammation of tissues inside the mouth and around the lips) can occur with chemotherapy. Eating becomes difficult. Brushing teeth causes bleeding and pain. Talking can be a problem because of sores inside the mouth. Kissing hurts, too. Feel free to set aside sensual activities involving the mouth for a while, including oral sex. Avoid foods high in acid because they may burn. Try a nonprescription pain reliever designed to relieve soreness in and around the mouth, such as Viscous Xylocaine.

Inflammation can also extend through your stomach and intestines. If severe, your physician may not allow you to eat for a few days to let your insides heal while you receive nutrients through a tube intravenously. If you have much nausea or vomiting during chemotherapy, ask your physician for help. Reduced appetite may cause weight loss, so keep foods available that are especially appealing to you.

Nausea hinders sex even more profoundly than fatigue. Take an antinausea medication about thirty minutes before starting sex. Try intercourse positions that keep your head upright to reduce queasiness. Avoid positions that put pressure on your abdomen. Women may not be able to give fellatio if it provokes nausea. Sometimes nipple stimulation produces nausea because of its hormone-releasing action on the pituitary gland. Take advantage of times when you feel better by having spontaneous sex. Spouses should understand that for a while you need to determine when to have sex.

Decreased resistance to infections.   Since chemotherapy alters your blood and can reduce the number of white blood cells, you can be more vulnerable to infections. Take precautions while on chemotherapy to avoid people with colds or other infections. Wash after shaking hands or touching doorknobs. Abstain from giving or receiving anal sex, because of its high potential for causing infection.

Vaginal intercourse is still permissible for most women receiving chemotherapy, although their husbands should thrust gently to prevent tearing or irritation. Occasionally a physician will ban intercourse for women at high risk for infection. Once immunity rebuilds after chemotherapy, they can return to their usual sexual activities. In the meantime, they should continue externally stimulated orgasms. In fact, it is wise to continue as much sexual activity as possible because sex increases circulation to the genitals and is psychologically beneficial when under stress. Douching is forbidden, though, because it creates an unnecessary opportunity for introducing germs into the vagina and can alter its natural acidity, making infections more likely.

Intercourse poses little risk for men undergoing chemotherapy as long as they avoid becoming infected. They should check the urinary opening on the penis for inflammation, and keep it away from their wives' anal area.

Both marital partners must remain monogamous to avoid bringing new germs into the closed sexual system they share. Germs that normally pose no threat can pass from a healthy person to someone in chemotherapy and cause bad infections while immunity is low.

Nerve changes. Sometimes chemotherapy, especially with repeated courses, affects sensory nerve function, causing numbness in the toes or fingertips. This problem is called "peripheral neuropathy," meaning the nerve endings don't work as well. Some people say they also have decreased sensation in the pelvis and that sexual stimulation doesn't seem as intense as usual. You may need stronger stimulation to reach orgasm. Take special care, however, not to irritate genital tissues. Use an artificial lubricant to decrease friction. Try a vibrator, but also increase other types of sexual stimulation that build arousal (erotic literature or videos, body caressing, nipple stimulation, etc.) so the genitals don't need stroking for as long to reach orgasm. Once treatment stops, normal sensations gradually return.

Changes in the genitals and reproductive organs. Women who haven't yet passed through menopause experience temporary shutdown of their ovaries with chemotherapy. Ovulation and menstruation stop. Estrogen and testosterone production decline. For a woman at about the age of menopause, this change may put her into permanent menopause. The breasts and the clitoris may shrink some. Estrogen replacement therapy is wise *if* it doesn't make the cancer worse.

In men, the testes may shut down, usually temporarily. If repeated chemotherapy is necessary, there is a small chance that they could cease functioning permanently. Sperm production declines. Testosterone production may or may not decrease. If it does drop, sex drive diminishes, as eventually will erectile ability if the depletion continues long-term. Testosterone replacement therapy is an option only if the cancer is of a type that testosterone does not promote. Usually the testes return to normal after chemotherapy stops.

If the wife is premenopausal, couples must use birth control while either partner is undergoing chemotherapy—even if the husband's sperm production is low. This is because chemotherapy may cause the sperm or ova to mutate, leading to serious DNA problems in the offspring. A woman must also avoid becoming pregnant while undergoing chemotherapy because the medicines used can be toxic to the baby or cause birth defects, especially during the first few months of gestation. Regardless of your gender, strongly consider banking your sperm or ova for the future before you start chemotherapy if there is any chance you might want more children from your own genes because, even after recovery, fertility may not return or you may cause birth defects.

Another genital problem is that chemotherapy can cause sores in the vagina. Women with breaks in the vaginal lining should abstain from intercourse until these areas have healed completely to avoid pain, irritation, development of larger areas of soreness, and infections. In the meantime, they ought to continue other sexual activities, such as external stimulation to orgasm.

Sex drive.   Not only may the side effects of chemotherapy deplete energy and cause testosterone decline in both men and women, there are also psychological reasons why someone with cancer may feel less interest in sex—anything from the crisis of illness to feelings of decreased self-worth to depression to loss of body image. Some experts say that rarely is decreased libido a problem with chemotherapy and, when it is, the reduction of sexual interest is temporary. Others say that sex drive declines more often than not, or that the effect lasts longer than the course of chemotherapy. The bottom line is that it's hard to pinpoint all the causes. Loss of sexual interest could be due to any of the mentioned possibilities and is probably due to multiple factors.

Therefore, look for answers everywhere you can. Try counseling—both for coming to terms with personal cancer issues and to explore sexual problems. Also, work with your physician to analyze your hormone levels, particularly testosterone. Do all you can to eliminate or decrease side effects that may hamper sexual interest. Consider the possibility of depression, because poor sex drive can be a symptom. Examine your marital relationship for tensions coming from your health crisis. Do whatever it takes and *don't give up without a fight*. Continued sexual function is very important to maintaining your feelings of being normal as you work through this time in your life.

Maybe you will be one of the fortunate couples who bypass serious sexual problems. Occasionally couples want sex even more when passing through the challenges of cancer.

> *You might think that this is odd, but Steven and I actually had sex more often during his cancer scare than usual. I guess we've always found that sex is comforting and strengthens our bond dur-*

ing a crisis. Maybe it's because sex is such a couple thing. It unites us in ways nothing else can. It's our way of saying that no matter what else goes wrong, our love is still strong and we're going to keep on acting as normal as we can.

Other Treatments for Cancer

It's hard not to become overly optimistic about new discoveries in the field of oncology. The research is coming from many angles, though, making it difficult to generalize about sexual implications. Let's briefly look at a few of the emerging therapies.

The first is immunotherapy, which stimulates the body's immune system to fight cancer with special white blood cells, called T-cells or B-cells, that attack cancer. So far complications with this approach seem only to cause flulike symptoms or rashes. No sexual side effects have yet come to our attention.

Most monoclonal antibodies, cancer vaccines, and gene therapies attacking the DNA of cancer cells are still experimental. No information about sexual side effects with these methods has become apparent because they're still under development or haven't been used on many patients. There is hope that cancer antibodies can be effective when cancer cell counts are at their lowest due to the action of other therapies.

Tamoxifen, a newly approved drug that helps prevent breast cancer, stops estrogen from binding with breast cells. Predominant side effects include blood clots, cataracts, and hot flashes. While it doesn't decrease estrogen or cause menopause, tamoxifen apparently disrupts the use of estrogen by various organs. Menopauselike symptoms, such as menstrual irregularities and spotting, vaginal dryness leading to irritation with intercourse, sleep disturbances from hot flashes causing emotional changes, and weight gain are some examples. Tamoxifen may also contribute to the development of uterine and liver cancer. It clearly is not a panacea. Only women who are at very high risk for breast cancer should consider taking it.

Herceptin is another new drug that helps to prolong the life of women who have metastatic breast cancer. It is a genetically engineered antibody that attacks the DNA of cancer cells, but it is useful in only about a third of breast cancer cases. Herceptin has fewer side effects than chemotherapy, primarily causing fever and chills (and heart problems rarely), but it has been available for too short a time for us to know about any sexual problems.

Winning the Battle Against Cancer

There are two battles to fight against cancer: the effect it has on your body and the effect it has on your spirit. Even if you lose the first battle, which is less likely than ever before, you will have failed if you allow cancer to kill your spirit. Keep your marriage in good repair, express your needs and fears to your spouse, and grip tightly to sexual expression of love. The challenges are great, but the victories are even greater. Don't let cancer rob you of sexual and marital happiness. You'll discover its power is nothing compared to the strength of your spirit.

9

THE TRUTH ABOUT SEX
AND HEART DISEASE

I was only forty-two years old when I became a member of that not-so-elite group of people with coronary disease. I know the cold, shaky sensation of fear that seizes the chest and squeezes the neck when angina heart pain hits. I struggle daily with blood pressure control and the exasperations of medication adjustments. I know what it's like to plan my funeral while waiting for cardiac catheterization. My intimate understanding of this disease extends back even further, though, to years spent as a coronary intensive-care nurse and my graduate school internship in cardiovascular surgery, never dreaming I would find my professional experience personally useful.

Coronary disease and high blood pressure are so common that they almost seem to be part of being human. If you live long enough, it's likely that you, too, will eventually develop a problem related to your cardiovascular system.

The impact of cardiovascular disease on sexual function can be profound. Not only does the buildup of cholesterol within blood vessels threaten erectile ability and block engorgement of the female genitals, but also medicines prescribed can sometimes inhibit sexual desire and erections. Heart attacks, congestive heart failure, coronary bypass surgery, dysrhythmias (irregular heartbeats), angina (heart pain), and other manifestations of cardiovascular disease each present threats to sexual activity for both men and women.

More limiting, though, is the fear factor. Anxiety about harming our hearts or risking death by participating in sex is responsible for more decline in sexual activity than any physical or pharmacological factor. Television and movies have distorted reality by filling our minds with scenes of lusty lovemaking when suddenly an actor grabs his chest and feigns death on the spot. Since chest pain accompanies heart attacks, we worry that even mild angina during sex indicates we've passed over the line of good sense and are about to play out our final scene in life, too.

These misconceptions seriously inhibit our ability to relax and to enjoy sex. Many men have sexual difficulty reestablishing sexual function following a heart attack, in spite of the fact that their erectile and other sexual problems are almost always caused by concerns about their hearts, not by the disease itself.

> *After my bypass surgery, one of my top five questions was "When can I start having sex again?" My doctor just said not to think about that yet and I never asked him again. I was scared spitless about trying, even after several months, when I was walking up to three miles a day. I just kept thinking, "What would happen to Ellen if I were to die on her right during a passionate moment?" She would probably die on the spot, too—of embarrassment at having to call the ambulance with me lying there naked.*

There are actually few occasions when it's necessary to stop sexual activity because of cardiovascular disease. These are during:

- severe episodes of congestive heart failure
- the first few weeks after a heart attack or bypass surgery
- the first few days after angioplasty or cardiac catheterization when exertion can provoke bleeding

Let's look at common cardiovascular disease conditions for ways to manage sexuality and alleviate fears.

HIGH BLOOD PRESSURE

High blood pressure (hypertension) occurs when the pressure of blood flowing through the vessels is consistently and significantly higher than normal. Often it happens without symptoms, so regular monitoring of blood pressure is important for everyone. Several factors contribute to hypertension, such as the blood volume being too great. Compare this to water pressure in your sink. If you slowly turn on the faucet, pressure of the water coming out is low. As you increase the volume of water flowing, water pressure increases as well. Sometimes kidney disease or other factors make our bodies retain fluid or sodium (which holds on to water), increasing blood volume and pressure.

Another cause of high blood pressure is narrowing of the inner diameter of arteries due to accumulation of cholesterol or atherosclerotic deposits. Sometimes arteries become more narrow from spasms or the action of nicotine. Whatever the cause, the heart has to work harder to push blood through, just as by twisting the nozzle of a garden hose to a smaller setting you dramatically increase the pressure of the water spray.

High blood pressure can be dangerous. Weakened places in the vascular (blood vessel) system rupture more easily under pressure, leading to a stroke if this occurs in the brain. Another effect is that the heart must work harder to get oxygen to distant body parts, causing it to enlarge over time, gradually decreasing its pumping effectiveness. Other dangers include heart attacks and damage to the kidneys.

Hypertension itself does not affect sexual function. Although blood pressure rises during sexual arousal, it also increases similarly during exercise, driving in heavy traffic, having an argument, becoming upset, or many other routine activities. Strokes do not occur more often during sexual activity. In fact, more happen during times of rest.

If hypertension is due to high cholesterol and generalized plaque deposits in the arteries, decreased blood flow to the genitals during sexual arousal may be a problem, though. One sign is that erections gradually become softer over the years because cholesterol builds up in pelvic arteries, as well as those to the heart and brain. For diagnosis, a man must undergo penile blood flow and pressure studies. Treatments include medications to improve blood pressure or to decrease cholesterol. Weight loss, exercise, stopping smoking, and dietary restriction of saturated fats may help over the long term. More drastic steps, such as surgery to remove deposits in the arteries to the penis or to bypass the blocked area to reestablish blood supply to the penis, are less common and have mixed results (see chapter 4 for more information).

Women generally don't lose as much sexual function from decreased blood flow to the pelvis. Even if they have less engorgement of the genitals, this doesn't prevent sexual arousal and orgasm. It may decrease vaginal lubrication, though—easily remedied by a generous application of a good water-soluble lubricant. Women do seem to have more headaches with elevated blood pressure, a distraction sometimes during sex when approaching orgasm. By controlling blood pressure through faithful compliance with prescribed medicines, reducing stress, and taking a nonprescription headache remedy before sex, hypertension headaches need not terminate a sex life. Intercourse positions that elevate the head help reduce headaches sometimes, too.

More often sexual problems related to hypertension are from the medications used to treat it. These same drugs are sometimes useful for other forms of cardiovascular disease as well and merit a closer look.

SEXUAL IMPLICATIONS OF MEDICATIONS USED TO TREAT CARDIOVASCULAR DISEASE

The danger in supplying information about medications for heart disease is that if you learn that one you're taking may affect sexual interest or performance, you might feel tempted to stop taking it. Physicians, nurses, and pharmacists often wonder whether it's wise to inform their clients about a medication's sexual side effects. The problem is not only that you might not take a medicine that you certainly need, thereby risking damage to yourself, but also you may be too embarrassed to confess your disregard of the doctor's prescription. Another risk of too much knowledge is that sometimes a side effect appears *because you expect it;* if you hadn't known it was a possibility, your mind wouldn't have succumbed to the placebo effect.

I ruined it for myself. I knew all about losing my potency from my friend Tom, who had been on blood pressure medicine for years, or at least I thought I did. I was really stupid, and started watching for it to happen in me, too. Sure enough, it did. I know now that by having just the tiniest expectation that the medication I was taking might change my erections, I became a victim of a self-fulfilling prophecy. I started to blame every little sexual glitch on the medicine and watched for signs of sexual problems so closely that I sabotaged my own goals.

It's extremely important whenever starting a new medication that you avoid thoughts about sexual side effects for a while. Give the medicine a fair chance to work for several weeks before looking for any possible signs of sexual difficulty. (Of course, if you have severe side effects earlier than that of any type, consult your physician.) If you've remained objective and have given the medicine a fair chance, but find it has significantly altered your interest in sex or the firmness of erections, speak up. Dosages and medications often need adjustment to best manage cardiovascular disease and side effects. Sexual problems are just as good reasons for making modifications in medicine as other difficulties are, so don't tell yourself (or let your physician tell you!) that this is just something you will have to learn to live with as part of the price for treating your disease.

Diuretics

Diuretics are medications that lower blood pressure by telling the kidneys to make more urine to get rid of extra fluid in circulation. There are many types of diuretics:

- furosemide (Lasix)
- spironolactone (Aldactone)
- hydrochlorothiazide (Diuril)
- chlorthalidone (Modiuretic)
- bumetanide (Bumex)
- triamterene (Dyrenium)
- metalazone (Zaroxolyn)
- and others

Since diuretics work by decreasing blood volume and lowering blood pressure, the hydraulic pressure necessary to produce an erection may become insufficient. Softer erections are an intolerable side effect worth reporting if intercourse becomes impossible.

Some diuretics cause potassium loss, leading to fatigue and muscle cramps that may affect sexual desire or performance. Cramps as "charley horses" seem to hit especially during sexual arousal and demand relief if sex is to continue. To combat low potassium, eat more oranges, bananas, and other foods high in

.

potassium, but also tell your physician about your symptoms because low potassium levels can cause dangerously irregular heartbeats.

ACE (Angiotensin Converting Enzyme) Inhibitors

ACE inhibitors are beneficial both for lowering blood pressure and for treating coronary disease. They act by blocking a hormone that stimulates blood vessel spasms and causes retention of water and sodium in the blood. Some ACE inhibitors are:

- enalapril (Vasotec)
- lisinopril (Prinivil)
- captopril (Capoten)
- ramipril (Altace)
- quinipril (Accupril)
- benazepril (Lotensin)
- and others

ACE inhibitors have their share of other side effects but seem to affect sexual performance less than diuretics do. Occasionally, as with any medicine that lowers blood pressure, erections may be more difficult to achieve because of decreased pressure in the vessels supplying the penis.

Digitalis

Digoxin (Lanoxin) is a digitalis preparation used for centuries to improve the effectiveness of the heart's pumping action. It's often prescribed for congestive heart failure because it slows the heart and helps it beat more strongly, making it also useful for certain rapid heart rate conditions. There are no sexual side effects to digitalis, although fatigue may affect sexual energy.

Alpha Blockers

Alpha blockers work by inhibiting the transmission of messages along certain nerve pathways that promote constriction of blood vessels. The result is that arteries relax and blood flows more easily at a lower pressure. Examples of alpha blockers are:

- doxazosin (Cardura)
- prazosin (Minipress)
- phentolamine (Regitine)
- clonidine (Catapres)
- terazosin (Hytrin)
- and others

Alpha blockers can reduce erectile function. Also, sometimes during physical exertion (such as sexual activity), a person on an alpha blocker experiences heart palpitations, a rapid heart rate, or an irregular heartbeat. These are not generally causes for concern but can be distracting.

Beta Blockers

Beta blockers stop the response of blood vessels and the heart to certain aspects of nerve stimulation. The result is a decreased heart rate and a lowered blood pressure. Beta blockers also affect the adrenal glands, inhibiting adrenaline release. Therefore, one common side effect is fatigue or loss of energy. Beta blockers include:

- propanolol (Inderal)
- acebutolol (Sectral)
- metoprolol (Lopressor)
- and others

Beta blockers can affect sexual function by decreasing sex drive, reducing erectile function, and limiting energy and vigor for any physical activity. If any of these symptoms severely alter your preferred sexual patterns, contact your physician for a medication adjustment.

Calcium Channel Blockers

Calcium channel blockers are effective in preventing angina and in reducing blood pressure. They seem to act by blocking the flow of calcium into muscle cells that control constriction of blood vessels, letting the vessels relax and dilate so blood can flow better to deliver more oxygen to the heart. Common calcium channel blockers are:

- nifedipine (Procardia, Adalat)
- verapamil (Isoptin)
- diltiazem hydrochloride (Tiazac, Cardizem)
- amlodipine (Norvasc)
- bepridil (Vascor)
- and others

As with all medication used to treat hypertension and heart disease, calcium channel blockers have some side effects. As far as sexual implications go, though, they are relatively unremarkable, unless the drop in blood pressure is dramatic enough to prevent constriction of penile blood vessels to trap blood for erection. Some people on calcium channel blockers notice during sexual arousal that their hearts beat more rapidly or that they have a feeling of flushing or heat in the face. Other than being a distraction, these phenomena are not problems and should not become excuses to stop having sex.

Nitrates

These medicines relax muscles in the walls of arteries throughout the body so the vessels can open wider, thereby decreasing blood pressure. However, they are more often used to treat angina because, when vessels supplying the heart open, oxygen flows through more easily. Examples of nitrates include:

- nitroglycerin (Nitrobid, Nitrostat)
- isosorbide mononitrate (Imdur)
- isosorbide dinitrate (Isorbid, Isordil)
- nitroprusside (Nitropress)
- and others

Since the effect of these vasodilators (medications that open the arteries) occurs throughout the body, not just in the heart, side effects can include headache and nasal congestion, but not usually any difficulties with sexual performance. In fact, letting a nitroglycerin pill dissolve under the tongue prior to sex helps prevent angina upon exertion. The headache and rapid heartbeat that nitroglycerin often stimulate disappear within minutes, certainly too soon to bother taking aspirin. Since the effect is so short-lived, the impact on sexual enjoyment need not be serious. The headaches caused by longer-acting nitrates usually appear predictably at about the same time every day, so avoid sex during those periods if your head hurts too much to let you relax.

An extremely important point to make regarding nitrates involves Viagra. Since Viagra also dilates blood vessels to improve blood flow, these drugs can compound each other's action to the point where undesirable and serious side effects appear. A man who is taking any form of a nitrate is not a candidate for Viagra. If he takes both, he risks a dramatic loss of blood pressure, fainting, and sudden cardiac death due to loss of adequate blood flow to the brain and the heart.

HEART ATTACK (MYOCARDIAL INFARCTION)

The primary goal of this section is to help those of you with heart disease—whether male or female—relinquish your fears about the safety of sex. Contrary to popular myth, sexual activity rarely causes death. Several studies confirm this, one of which, published in the *Journal of the American Medical Association*, reported that while having sex, people with heart disease temporarily increase the chance of having a heart attack from one in a hundred thousand to only two in a hundred thousand. The risk does not go up at all among people who exercise regularly.

Another study, published several years ago, has become a classic reference regarding death during sex. A pathologist found that out of more than fifty-five hundred cases of sudden death not due to violence that he studied, only 0.6 percent were related to sexual activity. Eighty percent of those few deaths that did occur happened during an extramarital affair. What these studies show is that the risk of having a heart attack or dying during sex is extremely low, even lower when sex takes place with a marital partner of many years, and yet lower again if a person exercises regularly. Heart attacks are much more likely to occur when you're under stress; exercising at a level much more exhausting than sex; or spontaneously, when a blood clot or a piece of cholesterol plaque breaks loose suddenly and plugs an artery.

This is not to say that once a person has had a heart attack there are no limitations at all on sexual activity. Common sense does dictate certain precautions. After all, a heart attack is by definition a life-threatening event that happens when a portion of the heart wall muscle dies from oxygen deprivation. If blood cannot flow through a vessel feeding the heart wall muscle because of blockage or spasms of an artery, oxygen deprivation appears as severe pain in the chest, neck, jaw, or left arm. Other signs of a heart attack include a feeling of pressure on the chest, nausea, vomiting, breaking into a sweat, difficulty breathing, and fainting.

Any time these warning signs appear, immediately call for medical assistance. Never wait, even if you aren't sure whether your pain is due to your heart or might simply be a case of bad heartburn. By delaying treatment the risk of death goes up dramatically, due to the onset of dangerous heart rhythms and the death of heart muscle. It's possible in many cases to reverse damage by dissolving a blood clot caught in a heart artery if treatment begins soon enough. For heart attacks due to blockage from cholesterol, an emergency cardiac catheterization or angioplasty (opening the narrowed section) may reestablish blood flow to the heart.

Hospitalization is mandatory following a heart attack. Before dismissal, your physician should discuss with you any temporary limitations on activities and line you up with a cardiac rehabilitation program. Prior to making a plan for resumption of activities, though, you will probably have a test within three weeks after your heart attack to assess how much function your heart now has. You will walk on a treadmill while an electrocardiogram (EKG) records the capacity of your heart to handle exercise. Another variation is a sonogram (echocardiogram), which bounces sound waves off your heart to give information about how effectively it functions. These tests are helpful not only for deciding how ready you are to resume tasks of daily living, but also for determining whether your treatment regimen is working well enough and how likely you are to have another heart attack. Be assured that exercise during a controlled test by a qualified physician is quite safe, even just a few days after a myocardial infarction (MI).

After a heart attack, people who can achieve a level of metabolism during exercise that reaches at least five "METs" are ready to begin cardiac rehabilitation and gradual progression of exercise at home. A MET is a unit of measurement that has to do with oxygen consumption at various levels of rest and activity. Sexual activity requires fewer than five METs if you use intercourse positions that don't tax your energy. The amount of stamina required for sexual arousal and orgasm, including intercourse, is much less than most people think. Of course, you can expend a considerable amount of energy at sex if you have intercourse standing up while bearing your spouse's entire weight, and thrusting rapidly for as long as you can possibly keep going! Acrobatic or athletic sexual techniques do indeed require great stamina, but aren't the type usually preferred by long-term sexual partners on a regular basis, and are certainly not necessary for sexual enjoyment during recovery from a heart attack.

Arousal and orgasm with intercourse while lying in bed with a spouse take about as much energy as climbing twenty steps at the rate of two steps per second. Many research studies verify that cozy, relaxed sex causes less strain on the heart than having an argument. Sex is not even as risky as simply getting up in the morning. Just getting out of bed after several hours of inactivity and sleep can alter blood pressure and loosen blood clots, causing a greater risk of an MI than having sex does.

There is a logical progression for resuming intercourse after a heart attack. First, abstain from all sexual activity for at least four weeks. This will allow the injured heart muscle to heal. During this time continue to maintain physical contact with your spouse, though, by hugging, holding, kissing, caressing, and giving each other massages. Avoid genital contact, though. Having an erection or feeling sexual arousal during the first month after a heart attack isn't dangerous, but ignore it until your heart has healed a while longer. When you can briskly climb twenty steps without angina, you are ready to resume sexual activity. Your physician can give you the medical clearance without having to try this at home alone, though, by doing the exercise testing at the hospital or medical office on a treadmill.

The next step is to bring yourself to orgasm while alone. The reason to start alone when resuming sex is not only because it's a less strenuous way to have an orgasm, it also can be a great confidence booster. By reaching orgasm without chest pain, controlled by you at your own pace, you'll be less afraid to try sex with your spouse.

You may notice, either during masturbation or with your spouse, that as you become more sexually aroused, your heart pounds or beats faster. Don't be concerned unless you start to have pain or feel faint, because these are normal manifestations of sexual arousal. You may find it helpful to cough a time or two if your heart starts beating irregularly or if you feel palpitations as you approach orgasm, because coughing stimulates a nerve that helps regulate heart rhythm. This little technique won't reduce the heart rate, though. If angina begins, signal your spouse and stop sexual activity for a minute or two. If the pain doesn't subside in a few seconds, take a nitroglycerin tablet and wait five minutes. When the pain lets up, you can continue. If the pain persists after taking two or three nitroglycerin tablets, contact your physician for further instructions.

Most people can safely resume full sexual activities, including intercourse, within four to eight weeks after an MI. If you are especially prone to angina, take a nitroglycerin tablet and have sex anyway. Don't feel obligated to perform in an active sexual role for three or four months, though. Stick to intercourse positions that allow the bed to support your entire weight. Let your spouse be on top, or use positions in which you both can recline on the bed (such as side-lying positions in which the man approaches the woman from behind for intercourse, or the woman lies on her back with her leg nearer the man over his hip as he faces her). As you increase other types of exercise, your tolerance for sexual activity will also improve. Anal intercourse is absolutely forbidden for six months after a heart attack, however, because it stimulates the vagus nerve, potentially causing a drop in heart rate and even cardiac arrest.

*Vince was pretty nervous about us starting to have sex again af-
ter my heart attack. I finally had to take him along on a visit to my
doctor so he could hear for himself that it was safe, as long as we
didn't try to set any records for endurance and we stuck to our favorite comfortable positions. Dr. Brown showed him my treadmill
EKG and how fast I was able to walk (a slow jog!) without any
trouble. Vince was still nervous the first time, but it didn't take
long for him to loosen up and start to enjoy himself.*

There are several ways by which you can avoid heart strain
and angina by simply avoiding sex at times when you are at
higher risk. For example, abstain right before or after participating in strenuous activity. Don't have sex when you are angry or
upset. Create a relaxed environment for sex. Make your bedroom
temperature comfortable—not too hot, cold, or humid. Avoid sex
soon after eating a large meal or drinking alcohol. Certainly stay
away from an extramarital affair because of the strain it puts on
the heart from excitement, nervousness, guilt, and the tendency
to use more lively sexual techniques.

If a rapid heart or breathing rate persists for more than twenty
minutes after intercourse, you may have overexerted. Other clues
to heart strain include palpitations or an irregular heartbeat lasting several minutes after orgasm. If you have trouble sleeping or
have extreme fatigue for up to a day after intercourse, consult
with your physician. Of course, any time chest pain appears and
persists in spite of nitroglycerin, get help immediately.

Congestive Heart Failure

Congestive heart failure (CHF) is what happens when blood flow
gets backed up because the heart isn't pumping effectively
enough to keep up with the workload. Fluid builds up in the body,
shown by weight gain, swelling in the feet and ankles, and increased fluid in and around the lungs. CHF often results from
years of high blood pressure that eventually take a toll on the
heart. Other factors can contribute as well, such as coronary
artery disease, a severe heart attack, heart valve problems, or inflammation of the heart. As CHF becomes worse, appetite disappears, extreme fatigue prevents all but the most essential activities,
and breathing becomes labored (especially while lying down). In

an acute episode, breathing becomes so difficult a person seriously fears for life.

> *My heart failure has been gradually getting worse over the past couple of years. I had to go to the emergency room three times during the night when it got really bad. Most of the time I manage pretty well, but I'd be lying if I didn't admit that it's put a crimp in our sex life. I don't feel I look as sexy when my ankles and feet puff up or when you can hear my breathing two rooms away. We used to be every weekenders at sex, but now we've learned that when I have a good day, we'd better take advantage of it because the weekend might not be so good. I'm just grateful Lou hasn't chucked it all, because I still get in the mood pretty often and know the day might come when I can't do much more than passively let him do all the work of lovemaking for both of us.*

Sex can continue with CHF as long as you are comfortable enough and interested. Physical activity does not worsen CHF and is quite beneficial for many reasons. Reduce your symptoms by restricting salt (sodium) and fluid intake, elevating your feet whenever possible, taking your medicines as prescribed, and staying away from all alcoholic drinks, because alcohol makes CHF worse. During acute episodes of CHF, no one with CHF is interested in doing anything except getting help to breathe more easily. The rest of the time, CHF primarily interferes with sexual function by making certain sexual intercourse positions more difficult. Positions that make breathing easier are those that keep the head and the shoulders elevated. Pad your bed's headboard with pillows or get a hospital-type bed so you can put your head up, allowing you to sit up somewhat during sex. Place blocks under the top of the bed or slip extra blankets under the head of the mattress. Some men with CHF find that having sex while sitting in a chair helps. A woman with CHF can straddle her husband, or recline against pillows crosswise in bed with her hips scooted to the edge of the mattress; her husband can then stand or kneel in front of her for intercourse with his hands on her knees for support and balance. The point is: experiment to find solutions. Conserving energy is important, too, so have sex when you're well rested, and use techniques that don't take much effort.

Coronary Bypass Surgery

Although surgery to place new vessels around the heart to better supply it with blood sounds like (and is) a serious procedure, there are few sexual implications. Prior to surgery, angina with exertion of any type (including sex) may be severe, but a few months after surgery, general health usually improves and endurance is better than ever.

As you recover from the operation, the chest incision and graft sites from where the new heart vessels were taken (usually one or both legs) will hurt and must heal. Postpone intercourse for at least four weeks, and follow the same gradual progressive regimen described for someone who has had a heart attack. Intercourse positions that avoid placing weight on the chest will prevent pain caused by contact with the incision. Expect your legs to hurt for up to three or four months, too, but be assured that the pain won't get worse during sex. General pain relievers will also make sex more comfortable.

> *I know surgical techniques have improved a lot since I had my triple bypass ten years ago, but I really suffered for quite a while afterward. When you think about it, it's no wonder, because to get to the heart they had to split open my breastbone, stop my heart from beating while they did the operation, and zap it to get it started again. My legs, where they took out the veins to use on my heart, ached for a long time, too. I wasn't in the mood for sex for at least three months. Between the pain and the worry about if I was sturdy enough for sex, I didn't even consider it. Carrie was patient, but made it clear that she was ready as soon as I was. We started off pretty shakily and I didn't have an erection until about the fourth month out, but we hung in there and sex is better than ever now.*

After healing is complete, sexual activity may be even more enjoyable than before the surgery. The improved oxygenation of your heart may permit you to try a wider variety of sexual styles. With relief from angina and breathing difficulties related to poor circulation to the heart, endurance does generally improve for all types of activities. As postoperative cardiac rehabilitation gradually increases your exercise tolerance, sexual activity can become more lively as well.

THE RULE OF THUMB

For each of the conditions described and other less common heart problems (heart valve disease, myocarditis, pacemaker implants, etc.), the important point to remember is that *by keeping sexual activity within the tolerance limits of your heart's capacity for exercise and by remaining faithful to your spouse, sex imposes very little risk.* If you can rapidly climb a tall flight of stairs (twenty steps), drive through heavy traffic for fifteen minutes, or have an argument without adverse symptoms, you can have leisurely sex with your spouse without difficulty. For more specific information about any exercise limits unique to your situation, talk to your physician or cardiac rehabilitation specialist.

10

STAYING SEXUAL
NO MATTER WHAT

We are susceptible to many other age-related sexual obstacles as new illnesses appear and old ones become more severe. This chapter will answer questions that people just like you have asked about challenges they faced, arranged alphabetically by topic.

AIDS

I'm sixty-three years old. Is it possible for me to get AIDS?

Absolutely! While it seems that this is a disease of the young, more and more older people are contracting the HIV virus and developing AIDS. The best protection is to stay sexually monogamous with your spouse. Even using a condom isn't very effective against HIV, contrary to the popular media message pushing condoms and "safe sex"—a misleading and dangerous concept. The virus is much smaller than the pores in the latex of the condom and can indeed pass from one person to another.

AGING

My wife and I are becoming more feeble. Are we too old and fragile for sex?

No. As long as nerve damage doesn't impair your ability to feel sexual stimulation, you both can still have orgasms until the end of life. Even if diabetes, a stroke, or other problem affects nerves, there are solutions. Since you do probably tire easily, though, release yourselves from the expectation that intercourse is the only way to have sex. Holding each other, cuddling, give genital caresses, and having occasional orgasms may constitute the perfect sex life in your case. When you do want intercourse, try having it in the morning, when you have more energy, and use positions that let you both lie down. Some couples use a water bed because the rocking motion assists thrusting. Talk with your wife about creative ways to survive sexually because sex is good for your health—physically, psychologically, and maritally.

ALZHEIMER'S DISEASE

My wife has Alzheimer's disease. How should I respond to her sexual overtures? I'm not even sure sometimes if she knows I'm her husband when she gets in these moods. Is it wrong of me to go ahead and have sex with her?

In a way, you are fortunate. Many people whose spouses have Alzheimer's disease lose interest in sex as their partners become more demanding, less rational, and (let's face it) exasperating. Caregiving activities and emotional stress threaten romance and sexual attraction. Often Alzheimer's disease changes the personality, making the affected person less inhibited or more insensitive to the healthy partner's feelings. It becomes more and more difficult to be interested in sex.

While many people with Alzheimer's gradually lose their libido, others become more outgoing sexually. At times their sexual drive seems too strong or inappropriately channeled. Some even make sexual advances to their children or strangers. There may be a tendency toward immodesty or public masturbation. Your wife may be convinced that you are cheating on her. She may often be unable to make lucid judgments, although she believes she is thinking clearly. These changes are symptoms of the disease and don't reflect what her true feelings would be if she were not under its power. An Alzheimer's disease support group for spouses will help you greatly.

To answer your question, feel free to respond positively to her sexual advances, and enjoy sex with her whenever you can. Even if she is confused about who you are, *you* know that you are her husband. *You* know that it is the disease making her confused, not a loss of her ordinarily good morals. The sexual activity is good for both of you physically, and can help relieve emotional tensions caused by the disease.

ARTHRITIS

All our lives, my husband and I have used the "missionary position" [man on top] for intercourse. For quite some time now, though, the arthritis in my hips has become so bad that it hurts to spread my legs. What can I do?

You are to be commended for not letting arthritis destroy your sexuality. It can threaten to do so in several ways. Many people find that chronic pain anywhere in the body is a distraction, and makes them feel so crabby and depressed that they lose interest in sex (and many other fun activities, too). If the arthritis leads to joint disfigurement, some people feel unattractive, imagining their spouses no longer want them. Men who take corticosteroids to reduce arthritic inflammation may have temporary erectile difficulty. Arthritis also makes many people tire more easily.

It often becomes harder for arthritic hips to separate wide enough for intercourse from the front without pain. You may have noticed that rotating your hip joints outward causes pain, too. Try to have sex during times when you are feeling more limber. Take your pain-relieving medicine at least thirty to sixty minutes before sex, soak in a tub of warm water, and stretch and move your legs from the hips in all directions before starting.

If these steps don't bring enough pain relief, it is time to give up old habits and use intercourse positions that allow you to keep your legs closer together. Try lying on your side with your back to your husband. Bend your knees up slightly and tilt your pelvis back toward him. This should expose your genitals from behind so he can enter your vagina. Place a pillow between your knees for even more comfort.

Another position is the "knee-chest," in which you are on your knees and forearms (or resting your head down on a pillow), with your bottom up in the air. Your husband kneels behind you, facing you for penile insertion. Experiment to find other positions that let you keep your legs closer together, too.

If it seems too calculating to plan sex for when you are feeling rested and having less pain, realize that sex can be fun even when it's not spontaneous. Use the time leading up to it for foreplay, romance, massage, and building your arousal. If your husband occasionally wants an impulsive "quickie" when you aren't feeling especially good, compromise by giving him oral sex in a position that is comfortable for you.

CIRCUMCISION

Our doctor has recommended a circumcision for my husband. At age seventy-eight, what purpose would that serve and what effect would it have?

It's my guess that your husband is either having a problem with phimosis (tightening of the foreskin around the head of the penis, dangerously cutting off circulation like a tourniquet) or balanitis (infection of the crown of the penis under the foreskin). A circumcision would cure both of these problems. The surgery carries little risk. His physician can use anesthesia that would let your husband sleep or remain awake during the procedure. He will be sore for a few weeks afterward, and penile stimulation must wait until healing is complete. After that, though, sex can resume as usual. Circumcision has no effect on sexual performance and does not, contrary to myth, cause premature ejaculation. Personal hygiene will be much easier, too.

DIABETES MELLITUS

I've had diabetes for almost thirty years—since I was a young woman. I still have a pretty good sex drive, but it seems that it's getting harder to feel anything "down there" anymore. Is my diabetes to blame?

Probably. As with men who have had diabetes for many years, the likelihood grows with time that some nerve damage will occur. Although you can't reverse it, you can enhance your orgasmic ability by asking your husband to spend more time caressing other parts of your body during foreplay. By building arousal that way you will need less clitoral stimulation for orgasm. Also, ask him to use more pressure on your clitoris or try using a vibrator to get stronger sensations, taking care not to injure your tissues. Inspect your genitals after sex for signs of irritation, since you are more prone to infection and delayed healing. Follow your physician's instructions for controlling your diabetes. That will do more than anything else to slow loss of genital sensations.

Special note to men with diabetes: For more information about the effects of diabetes on men, see chapter 4.

Heartburn

The older I get, the worse my heartburn is during sex. What can I do?

There are several reasons why your heartburn may be worsening. Aging muscles at the bottom of your esophagus loosen and may not work as well to keep acid in the stomach. You may have developed a hiatal hernia. Extra weight you've gained over the years may be pressing against your stomach when you lie down, forcing acid into your esophagus. There are other possibilities, too. See your physician for diagnosis and treatment, including a prescription for one of the excellent medicines now available for reducing "gastric reflux." In the meantime, don't eat or drink for an hour (two hours, if possible) before sex. Take an antacid before starting, then lie on your left side for a minute or two until you burp up any air bubbles sitting in your stomach. Then prop up your head and shoulders with pillows, or have sex in positions that allow you to stay upright.

Hip Replacement

My doctor has recommended that I have a "total hip arthroplasty," a replacement of my entire hip joint. How will this affect my ability to have intercourse with my husband?

You probably already have many more problems enjoying sex right now than you will if you proceed with the operation. Before surgery, most people with hip disease have sexual difficulty because of pain and limited movement. Wait a couple of months after surgery before having intercourse again, although you can resume clitoral stimulation right away. Your surgeon may recommend that you permanently avoid intercourse positions that require you to spread your knees farther apart than twenty-four inches, but don't let that stop you from having sex within that limit using other positions. Once healing is complete, your sex life will probably improve dramatically and you will be glad you had the surgery.

MULTIPLE SCLEROSIS

My husband has had multiple sclerosis for almost ten years. He is definitely losing erectile function but doesn't seem to be bothered by it. Is this normal?

About half of people with multiple sclerosis (MS) have some sexual dysfunction. Male complaints include loss of sex drive, premature ejaculation, decreased sensation in the penis, difficulty having erections, or delayed or blocked orgasms. Testosterone levels may also drop as a result of poor nerve stimulation of the testes with advancing MS. Women with MS are more likely to have decreased sensations in the clitoris and vagina, poorer vaginal lubrication, difficulty reaching orgasm, or a decline in libido. Both sexes are susceptible to muscle spasticity and urine leakage during sexual arousal. These problems are primarily due to the effects of MS on nerves, and become more severe as time passes. Sexual problems are more often due to neurological deterioration caused by the MS rather than psychological problems. However, brain degeneration sometimes causes memory loss, disappearance of all sexual interest, difficulty learning new things, and even mental illness.

While sexual problems vary in severity, people with MS usually view their other problems related to loss of coordination and mobility to be more important than sexual dysfunctions. This, along with some possible loss of brain function, may explain why your husband doesn't seem as concerned about his declining sexual performance as you are. Unfortunately, there is no way to reverse neurologic damage. Your best recourse is to talk frankly to your husband about your concerns in a manner that presents it as a need *you* have, not as a problem *he* has. Tell him your interest in sex is still strong and you're wondering if he would be willing to try Viagra, penile injections to produce erections, or a penile implant. Bring up the subject together at his next doctor's visit.

If he isn't willing to get help, you must redefine for yourself what shape you want your own sex life to take as you adapt to his gradual sexual retreat. Take advantage of those times when he shows interest, express your appreciation for him, and savor those moments. Continue to love him and express your affection to him physically. You must also take responsibility for your own sexual happiness, though. Give yourself permission to explore the pleasures of masturbation, and use a dildo to keep your vagina open and healthy.

Special note to women with MS: Loss of sensation to the genitals can be counteracted somewhat by using stronger stimulation, but inspect the genitals carefully after sex to be sure they are not becoming irritated. Use a liberal amount of artificial lubricant as well. Specific suggestions in chapter 3 for problems with loss of sex drive may help, too.

NURSING HOME RIGHTS

My mother and I recently had to place Dad in a nursing home because he needs constant care. His mind is sharp, though, so it was an agonizing decision. He's now asking why he and Mom can't have some privacy for a little "hanky-panky" when she visits. The nursing home staff says that for safety reasons doors must remain open unless an aide is in the room. Mom is too nervous to try anything anyway because there are no locks on the doors. What should we do?

Entering a nursing home does not mean relinquishing rights to privacy, sexual intimacy, and conjugal visits by a spouse. Your father has a legal right to a lock on his door and to have time alone with your mother, as long as they both understand that the staff has a key in case of emergency. His nurse call button is readily available should they need help, too. If he has a roommate, the facility should provide a private room for conjugal visits. Even better, arrange for him to have a pass to come home occasionally if possible. It does take effort, but he and your mother would be much more comfortable and greatly appreciative. They need each other now more than ever, and it is your duty to be an advocate for their rights. If the nursing home refuses to cooperate, ask the physician to write an order for conjugal visits, see an attorney, or transfer your father to a different facility.

PARKINSON'S DISEASE

My husband has Parkinsonism. He has been amazingly resilient and adaptable in spite of the problems it has caused. Lately, though, he has been showing signs of depression and is becoming very frus-

trated about his medicine not controlling his tremors well enough. Our sex life is starting to decline, but is it due to the disease or the depression?

It could be due to either factor or both. If your husband is becoming discouraged, losing self-confidence, and feeling embarrassed about the tremors, he may well experience a loss of sex drive or erectile dysfunction. He may see the worsening of his condition as a reason to grieve; his plans for his later years are being ruined by the fatigue and loss of mobility to which he is now more vulnerable. He may feel as if he is letting you down. Perhaps loss of urinary control is a source of embarrassment to him that challenges his feelings of masculinity. The solutions to depression are to talk out issues between yourselves and to get professional counseling, if necessary. You must establish a healthy pattern of communication and adjustment now, because as his disease progresses you will face even more challenges.

Parkinsonism can also physically affect sexual function by lowering sex drive, causing premature ejaculation, or interfering with erection. With advancing loss of muscle control, intercourse can be more difficult due to tremors or muscle rigidity, especially when he is tired. Another possible cause is dopamine, a medicine he may be taking that can contribute to depression. Ask his physician about alternatives.

Shift your sexual patterns to early in the day, when he is more rested. Take advantage of times when his tremors aren't as severe. Experiment with positions to identify those that make the tremors worse. Try heat and massage to relax tremors and rigidity. Explore sexual stimulation of other erogenous zones to enhance arousal without genital focus. If he is having trouble with erections and if his health otherwise is quite good, investigate other options for producing erections (see chapter 5).

Special note to women with Parkinsonism: In addition to the challenges listed above, you are also more prone to loss of orgasmic function. Before deciding that the problem is irreversible, try the suggestions in chapter 4. If you do permanently lose your ability to orgasm, you retain the capacity to participate in intercourse. Give your husband this gift gladly. Be sure to use plenty of lubricant and enjoy the pleasure he receives, as well as knowing that he still wants you. Soak up the warmth of physical contact and intimacy. Encourage him to explore other parts of your body for sensitive areas that may respond sexually to his touch and kiss, even to the point of orgasm.

PEYRONIE'S DISEASE

As I get older, my penis is becoming more curved and recently has started taking on a twisted appearance during erections. Is this normal?

I assume you are not talking about a tendency of your penis to angle to the right or the left, which is a normal phenomenon. Because of the twisted shape you describe, you probably have Peyronie's disease. The inner lining of one of your corpora cavernosa has developed plaques or is becoming fibrotic due to an injury to your penis, or perhaps due to a hereditary factor. You may be able to feel the fibrosis while your penis is soft as a lump or thickened area about a quarter inch under the skin. Fibrous tissue doesn't stretch and expand as well as normal tissue during engorgement and erection; therefore your penis tends to bend or twist in the direction of the fibrosis. The condition may gradually diminish, although it often worsens with age. As long as it causes you no pain, does not make your penis lose sensation, and as long as you can still have intercourse, there is no cause for concern. If you find that the problem is becoming severe, surgery to release the fibrosis is an option. It's very important that you seek the help of a qualified sex therapist if you find that your condition is causing you so much psychological trauma that you are having difficulty achieving erections at all.

SPINAL CORD INJURY

My husband fell off a ladder while painting the house a few months ago and broke his back. He has permanent spinal cord damage. Recently he hinted that he wants to resume our sex life. I thought that people with spinal cord injuries could no longer have sex. Is he kidding himself? What should I do?

The simplest answer is that, as long as a person is not in a coma and wants sex, sexuality need never end. This doesn't mean it will never need some adjustments, though. Now is one of those times calling for some big adjustments. To understand what your husband is capable of sexually, let's review some basic neurology.

The spinal cord serves three primary purposes: (1) to carry messages from the body to the brain, telling it that it feels something; (2) to carry messages from the brain to the body, telling muscles to move; and (3) to signal various muscles to respond to stimulation automatically by reflex action without involving the brain. To determine how much sexual function your husband has, it is necessary to know where along the spinal cord his injury occurred and whether the injury completely interrupted nerve messages at that level, or whether some messages can still get through.

If the injury was incomplete, your husband's brain may still be able to control some muscles by sending messages through the spinal cord. He may still be able to feel some sensations. If he can consciously squeeze his rectal muscles, he may have some genital function. If the injury is complete, though, there is probably permanent paralysis and loss of sensation below that level of the spinal cord. Affected muscles are flaccid or limp at first, but later can become stiff or spastic, especially if reflexes below the level of the injury remain intact. If spasms inhibit intercourse or become a severe distraction, experiment with positions that may not provoke the spasms so severely. Also, ask his physician for a medication that reduces spasms without altering genital function.

As long as the reflex arc responsible for erections brought on automatically by physical contact with the penis remain functional, your husband may have erections when you touch his penis, because reflexes work without nerve messages traveling to the brain. If his injury was complete, though, he won't have erections simply by thinking about or watching sex—that would require getting messages from the brain. Just because a man has penile engorgement when his erection reflex is still working doesn't mean that he can feel penile stimulation. It is possible that you could stimulate him to erection manually and be able to have intercourse briefly before the erection subsides. Usually reflex erections don't last long, though. Viagra may help in these situations.

Therefore, you may want to discuss with him other ways to

maintain an erection for intercourse—*if* intercourse is important to you. Several methods described in chapter 4 will work: vacuum devices, constriction bands, a penile implant, penile injections, or medicine pellets inserted into his urinary opening. Even Viagra is successful in some cases of spinal cord injury. Since he probably has little genital sensation (if any), you will have to be actively involved in making these methods work (especially if he doesn't have the use of his arms). Take responsibility for inspecting his penis afterward. Get medical attention for him if you see any problems or if his erections don't subside within an hour or so. You can also learn how to stimulate your husband's prostate to produce an erection: put on a latex glove, lubricate the finger you'll use, gently push it about three inches into his rectum, and massage the front wall (the side toward his abdomen). Regardless of how he gets an erection, you'll need to provide the thrusting movement for intercourse, since he probably has limited use of his hips, if any. Try different positions to find those that work best.

Erection, orgasm, and ejaculation are all separate entities in terms of nerve control. If your husband can have an erection, he may not necessarily be able to have an orgasm, or, if he can, he may not feel that it's happening. Some men have orgasms without erections. Many with spinal cord injuries lose the ability to ejaculate externally (orgasm pushes the semen into the bladder, called "retrograde ejaculation").

You may wonder what to do about his bladder and bowel function during sex. If he wears a urinary catheter at all times, you can just bend it back along the shaft of his penis, or remove it if you know or if he knows how to reinsert it later. If he doesn't use a catheter, he should empty his bladder before sex. Once erect, he shouldn't be able to leak urine. Take advantage of opportunities to have sex soon after his bowel movements or administer an enema first to prevent an accident.

For couples interested in getting pregnant, a physician may be able to produce ejaculation through mild electrical stimulation of the prostate or penis. Even with retrograde ejaculation, sperm can be drained from the bladder for artificial insemination. These methods work best within the first few months after injury, because the number of sperm gradually drops, and those made are less active.

For the sake of discussion, let's say that your husband has entirely lost all ability to have erections and cannot feel any genital sensations. How can you have a sex life under these conditions? You both must decide that you will learn new ways of being sexual. Even if your husband's injury is at the cervical (neck) level, he still can function as a sexual being. He can enjoy sex in at least three ways: (1) mentally through imagery, reading, watching videos, looking at your body, and so forth; (2) by enjoying the sensations he has in the parts of his body that he can still feel; and (3) by giving you sexual pleasure. Grant yourselves permission to explore every square inch of his skin that still has sensation. The portion of his body that can still perceive touch is the area with which you have to work. Pay special attention to known erogenous zones (earlobes, neck, inside of the mouth, the nipples, the armpits, etc.). One area that people with spinal cord injuries say seems to be especially sensitive to touch is the line of demarcation at which the injury occurred. The skin at this line between sensation and numbness may respond to sexual stimulation. By touching, massaging, licking, sucking, blowing on it, or any other techniques you want to try, you may be able to help your husband learn how to orgasm again using his nongenital body parts. As incredible as this may sound, many people have succeeded in doing just that.

He can also be an active participant in sex by giving you sexual enjoyment. If he can use his arms or hands, he can manually stimulate your clitoris or insert a finger or a dildo into your vagina to simulate intercourse. If he only has use of his head, he still can use his tongue and lips to excite your clitoris if you are willing to place your genitals close to his mouth. Feel free to rub your clitoris on his body to bring yourself to orgasm while he watches.

Your attitude is extremely important to your husband. Don't expect his interest in sex to disappear just because he had a spinal cord injury. He probably cares a great deal about your sexual happiness. Undoubtedly you perform many tasks for him and have altered your life because of his limitations. Allow him to do something nice for you now, too. He needs to contribute to the relationship. Most older people who have had spinal cord injuries for many years report that they generally feel quite healthy and rank the quality of their lives as good or excellent. An important part of this is sexual fulfillment.

Special note to women with spinal cord injuries: Intercourse remains possible as a more passive participant, but your husband should check your vagina for adequate lubrication and use an artificial lubricant if needed. Some women retain their ability to lubricate as a reflex of genital stimulation, whether they can feel the contact or not. Others can still lubricate from psychological sexual stimulation if some nerve messages can get through the injured area of the spine from the brain. The ability to feel genital sensations and have orgasms depends on whether the damage completely impaired all nerve pathways at the level of the injury. Refer to the information above about how to learn to orgasm in new ways. Women with spinal cord injuries remain fertile until menopause, although their menstrual periods may be irregular, so be sure to use birth control unless you want to get pregnant or are past menopause.

STROKE

My husband just had a stroke. Will we be able to have sex anymore?

The general answer is yes, you probably can. To better understand your chances, it's important to know how the cerebrovascular accident (CVA or stroke) has affected him and how much function he will regain. Don't expect to be able to predict that based on what he can do today, though. Recovery takes time. He may lose sensation to one side of his body or certain parts of his body; he may lose voluntary muscle control but not necessarily lose sensation; the area of his brain contributing to sex drive may be damaged; or his speech or sight may be altered. Any function lost may return. It is the responsibility of your husband's physician to explain what to expect, including the changes affecting sexual function. Let's go over ways in which you can adapt.

If your husband has become permanently paralyzed on one side, push the bed against the wall, keeping him between you and the wall to prevent him from falling. Select intercourse positions that help him keep his balance, using pillows to prop his weaker side in place. Consider having hand grips installed on your bed's headboard, or have a "trapeze" placed over your bed (a bar or ring that dangles within reach over the bed for him to hang on to when he wants to sit up or turn).

Your husband will probably be weak for several weeks or

months, so expect to do most of the thrusting during intercourse yourself. You may both find it easier to stick to manual stimulation or oral sex for a while.

Permanent paralysis can turn into spasticity during sexual arousal—a rigidity or uncontrollable tremoring in the affected limbs. Try not to let spasms interrupt your sexual focus. Your husband may eventually be able to control spasms somewhat by using medications his physician prescribes, and by exercise, even passively putting the paralyzed muscles through a range of movements before sex to loosen the muscles some. Passive exercise in which he or someone else actually lifts, pushes, and pulls each paralyzed joint through its full extent of movement several times each day will also prevent contractures (freezing of joints into curled-up positions). Contractures make some sexual positions difficult, if not impossible.

If your husband loses the sense of touch in certain areas, you will need to adjust your sexual stimulation techniques. Spend more time building sexual arousal by focusing on parts of his body that are still sensitive. Expect him to have trouble for a while identifying where you are touching him, a typical after-effect of a stroke. Approach him from his active side. This will also help if he loses sight in half of his vision from the stroke and cannot see you if you are on his blinded side.

For several weeks and perhaps longer, your husband may have trouble controlling his urine and bowel movements. Remind him to empty his bladder and bowel before starting sex, because arousal can stimulate activity in these organs. Treat accidents as an expected event, doing everything possible not to make him feel more ashamed than he probably will anyway.

Many other possible coexisting factors compound sexual challenges: hypertension, medication side effects, diabetes, cardiovascular disease, and so forth. Some men experience declining testosterone levels if nerve supply to the testes was compromised. Some men lose the ability to ejaculate after a stroke, but not necessarily the ability to orgasm, so don't make any assumptions, and explore all the possibilities.

Your husband will probably experience anger, grief, and loss of self-confidence for a while. A stroke is a frightening blow to his self-image and his view of the future, particularly if full function doesn't return. He may feel humiliated if he needs help eating, drools uncontrollably, or if his appearance changes because of drooping facial muscles. You will play a key role in helping him feel masculine, important, loved, wanted, and needed as he recovers. If you see signs of prolonged or deepening depression, get professional help for him. If he loses the ability to speak or has difficulty speaking, that will be a special challenge to his ability to communicate with you and to talk out his feelings. Suggest that he becomes part of a support group. If he can still write, buy a journal for him to record his thoughts as he works through his feelings. Don't be surprised if sex isn't on his mind for several weeks. Some men wonder first about whether sexual function will return, while others focus entirely on walking, talking, reestablishing routines, and other concerns.

There are times when strokes affect people even more profoundly. They lose their ability to think clearly, reason, remember, and communicate thoughts. If your husband has trouble understanding that you want sex or telling you that *he* wants sex, you must decide to have the patience of Job. Try communicating in new ways. Repeat your messages. Wait a while and try again. Take him to a different room, turn on the lights, or alter your environment in other ways that help him to refocus. Try singing your message, because music communicates to a different part of the brain than spoken words do. He may be able to sing his message to you more easily, too.

If his stroke was in the right side of the brain, he may have altered judgment and become more impulsive. He may unintentionally skip foreplay and start with intercourse, because he has lost the ability to put steps in the right order. Give him simple directions and positive feedback. If his stroke occurred on the left side of his brain, he may seem to be moving in slow motion, with uncertain movements. His personality may be more cautious than it used to be, so give him reassurance and encouragement, especially if he shies away from trying sex.

You, too, will need support. Since strokes can cause death, you've probably had a terrible scare. Perhaps you'll find that your husband now totally focuses on his own needs and that you have to start becoming responsible for your personal happiness—sexually and otherwise. If you have to take on a caregiver role, review the suggestions in chapter 8 for sexual adjustment.

If your husband recovers enough to return home after his stroke, there is definitely a sexual future for you together. A critical factor will be whether he is willing to go through "sexual rehabilitation" along with his speech, physical, or occupational therapy. Sexual rehabilitation consists of working with you to discover what types of genital function he still has, solving problems introduced by limited mobility or lost sensation, having patience as you both adjust to possible cognitive changes in his brain, and sex therapy if he has psychological barriers caused by his altered self-image.

Weight Gain

My wife and I have both put on several pounds as we got older. What can we do to make sex more comfortable for us?

Weight gain affects sexual activity in several ways. You may be unable to thrust as long without getting tired. Penile penetration may be too shallow if your tummy is very large. You may have lost feelings of sexual attractiveness if you buy into the myth that only the thin are sexy. Your muscles and joints could have trouble supporting your weight in some intercourse positions. You may have trouble breathing when lying flat in bed. Your weight may be too much for your wife to breathe easily if you use the man-on-top method.

None of these problems is insurmountable, though. Use pillows for support or to allow you to sit up more. If you have a large tub or a swimming pool, have sex in the water to buoy up your weight. A water bed can help, too. Have intercourse in positions that avoid belly-to-belly contact, such as:

- you approach your wife's vagina from behind ("rear entry"— not to be confused with anal intercourse!)
- your wife straddles you on her knees and remains upright
- your wife lies on her back with you on your side facing her, putting her leg nearer you over your hip
- your wife scootches her hips to the edge of the side of the bed and brings her knees back; you stand at the edge of the bed and thrust while balancing your hands on her knees

Keep a sense of humor about your maturing physiques and explore new techniques that accommodate your needs.

CONCLUSION

Sexual survival depends on you—your willingness to learn, grow, communicate, experiment, adapt, and stay committed. As long as you can love, you are still a sexual person with much to give and to get. Don't let that part of you die.

BIBLIOGRAPHY

Chapter 1
Martin, Clyde. 1977. "Sexual Activity in the Ageing Male." In *Handbook of Sexology*. Edited by John Money and H. Musaph. New York: Elsevier/North Holland Biomedical Press.
Masters, William. 1986. "Sex and Aging—Expectations and Reality." *Hospital Practice* 21:175–198.
Michael, Robert, John Gagnon, Edward Laumann, and Gina Kolata. 1994. *Sex in America: A Definitive Study*. Boston: Little, Brown.
Pfeiffer, Eric, and G. C. Davis. 1972. "Determinants of Sexual Behavior in Middle and Old Age." *Journal of the American Geriatrics Society* 20:151–158.
Zilbergeld, Bernie. 1982. "Is There Sex after the Honeymoon?" The Changing Family Conference, Iowa City, Iowa, February 19.

Chapter 2
Comfort, Alex. 1972. *Joy of Sex*. New York: Simon & Schuster.
Hite, Shere. 1976. *The Hite Report: A Nationwide Study of Female Sexuality*. New York: Dell.
Masters, William, and Virginia Johnson. 1966. *Human Sexual Response*. Boston: Little, Brown.
Pfeiffer, Eric, and G. C. Davis, 1972. "Determinants of Sexual Behavior in Middle and Old Age." *Journal of the American Geriatrics Society* 20:151–158.
Weindruch, Rick. 1996. "The Retardation of Aging by Calorie Restriction: Studies in Rodents and Primates." *Toxicologic Pathology* 24:742–745.

Chapter 3
Barbach, Lonnie. 1975. *For Yourself: The Fulfillment of Female Sexuality*. Garden City, N.Y.: Doubleday.
Burns, David. 1980. *Feeling Good: The New Mood Therapy*. New York: William Morrow.

Chapter 4
Burns, David. 1980. *Feeling Good: The New Mood Therapy*. New York: William Morrow.
Pfizer, Incorporated. 1998. *Viagra in Perspective*. New York: Pfizer Incorporated.

Chapter 7

Arcangeli, C. G., D. K. Ornstein, D. W. Keetch, and G. L. Andriole. 1997. "Prostate-Specific Antigen as a Screening Test for Prostate Cancer." *Urologic Clinics of North America* 24:299–314.

Landis, Sarah, Taylor Murray, Sherry Bolden, and Phyllis Wingo. 1998. "Cancer Statistics, 1998." *CA: Cancer Journal for Clinicians* 48:6–29.

Partin, A. W., and H. B. Carter, 1996. "The Use of Prostate-Specific Antigen and Free/Total Prostate-Specific Antigen in the Diagnosis of Localized Prostate Cancer." *Urologic Clinics of North America* 23:531–540.

Chapter 9

Muller, James, Murray Mittlemann, Malcolm Maclure, Jane Sherwood, and Geoffrey Tofler. 1996. "Triggering Myocardial Infarction by Sexual Activity: Low Absolute Risk and Prevention by Regular Physical Exertion." *Journal of the American Medical Association* 275:1405–1409.

Ueno, M. 1963. "The So-Called Coition Death." *Japanese Journal of Legal Medicine* 17:330–340.

INDEX

ABOUT THE AUTHOR

Marvel L. Williamson, Ph.D., R.N., began teaching what she knew about sex in the fourth grade to her wide-eyed classmates and has been opening eyes ever since. Before becoming a sexologist, her nursing experience included coronary care, gynecology, surgery, intensive care, the burn unit, labor and delivery, and general adult health. In 1981 she received her sexology certification from the American Association of Sex Educators, Counselors, and Therapists. She was an assistant professor of nursing and sexuality for the Colleges of Nursing, Medicine, and Liberal Arts at the University of Iowa until 1991. She has also taught sexuality at the University of Kansas School of Medicine and the Southwest Georgia Family Practice Residency. Dr. Williamson is the former director of the School of Nursing at Park University in Kansas City, Missouri, and is now a sexologist in the Washington, D.C., area. Her sex research has been published in many professional journals and has appeared in the *New York Times*, *Glamour Magazine*, *AMA News*, *American Baby*, *Prevention Magazine*, numerous local and regional newspapers, on CNN, on many local news and talk shows, and on National Public Radio. She has an extensive record as a featured speaker on sexuality to both lay and professional groups. Dr. Williamson has been married to Paul Williamson, M.D., for more than twenty-five years. They have two sons, Marcus and Sean.